WHAT YOU MUST KNOW ABOUT
FOOD AND SUPPLEMENTS FOR OPTIMAL VISION CARE

JEFFREY ANSHEL, OD

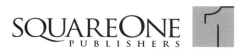

SQUAREONE
PUBLISHERS

EDITOR: Michael Weatherhead
COVER DESIGNER: Jeannie Tudor
TYPESETTER: Gary A. Rosenberg

The information and advice contained in this book are based upon the research and the personal and professional experiences of the authors. They are not intended as a substitute for consulting with a health care professional. The publisher and authors are not responsible for any adverse effects or consequences resulting from the use of any of the suggestions, preparations, or procedures discussed in this book. All matters pertaining to your physical health should be supervised by a health care professional. It is a sign of wisdom, not cowardice, to seek a second or third opinion.

Square One Publishers
115 Herricks Road
Garden City Park, NY 11040
(516) 535-2010 • (877) 900-BOOK
www.squareonepublishers.com

Library of Congress Cataloging-in-Publication Data

Anshel, Jeffrey.
  What you must know about food and supplements for optimal vision care / Jeffrey Anshel, OD.
      pages cm
    ISBN 978-0-7570-0410-0
  1. Eye—Diseases—Nutritional aspects—Popular works. 2. Eye—Care and hygiene—Popular works. 3. Self-care, Health—Popular works. I. Title.
    RE51.A634 2015
    617.7—dc23
                              2015006306

Copyright © 2015 by Jeffrey Anshel

All rights reserved. No part of this publication may be reproduced, stored in a retrieval system, or transmitted, in any form or by any means, electronic, mechanical, photocopying, recording, or otherwise, without the prior written permission of the publisher.

Printed in the United States of America

10   9   8   7   6   5   4   3   2   1

Contents

Part Three NUTRITIONAL APPROACHES

Acknowledgments

No comprehensive text can be effectively written by one person. Over the course of writing this book, I had the honor of working with some very intelligent, dedicated, and fascinating people, many of whom graciously offered assistance in proofreading and reviewing this material at every turn. A special thanks to Ellen Troyer, MT, MA, chief research officer and CEO of Biosyntrx, Inc., who has been a mentor to me during my nutritional education. She took time out of her busy and demanding schedule to review the section on nutrition and vision.

Thanks to Brian Banks of Natural Ophthalmics for his confidence in me and for reviewing the section on homeopathy. Dr. A. Paul Chous is a national speaker and expert in diabetes who has also been very generous in his support of my work. His contributions to the information on diabetes are greatly appreciated. Special recognition goes to Dr. Stuart Richer, who has been a good friend and ardent supporter of my mission to educate doctors in nutrition. Stuart has always challenged me to exceed my limitations and think outside the box. His belief in the need for this book was invaluable. I would also like to thank the members of the Ocular Nutrition Society, who are hungry for knowledge concerning nutritional approaches to vision disorders.

This book represents the combined efforts of a number of helpful experts whose commitment and knowledge were required for its message to be expressed effectively. I thank them all again for their dedication.

Of course, I would like to thank my friends and family members, who continue to support my personal and professional goals.

Preface

After graduating optometry school in 1975 and spending two years practicing in the US Navy, I opened a practice of optometry at the Holistic Healing Arts clinic in Solana Beach, California. The idea of holistic healing was a New Age concept that referred to healing using the body, mind, and spirit. This clinic had a wide array of practitioners, including acupuncturists, chiropractors, nutritionists, physical therapists, massage therapists, and homeopaths. These practitioners included nutrition as a part of their protocols. My idea of holistic optometry was grounded in the fact that I was offering vision therapy, which included not only helping kids with reading and learning problems, but also teaching them basic techniques to improve their vision. I wanted to include everything in my approach to the treatment of vision problems. Unfortunately, there were few optometric courses offering nutritional education. This area was foreign to the profession. I learned some of the basics of nutrition and applied them to my own life.

In 2001, the findings of the AREDS study were released, suggesting that nutrition might slow progression of age-related macular degeneration. The industry was abuzz with this new information, and speakers at conferences started talking about how wonderful the study's formula was and why we should be recommending it. But I felt that there was more to it.

A few years later, I realized there was quite a bit of stretching of the truth regarding the role of nutrition in eye health, and that much of it was geared to sell products. I felt the industry needed an independent source of research on ocular nutrition. I consulted with a few colleagues and we created the Ocular Nutrition Society in 2008. During this time, I had intermittently been working on a book that would eventually be published as *Smart Medicine for Your Eyes*. Recently, I decided to revise that book, turning it into this user-friendly guide.

Introduction

Eyecare professionals are committed to giving each patient a lifetime of seeing clearly and comfortably with healthy eyes. They draw upon their educations and years of experience to assist in the remediation of eye health and the treatment of vision disorders. I have had the fortune of exploring several modalities of healthcare, ranging from Eastern philosophies to ancient European concepts. What I have learned is that there may be more than one truth when it comes to healing the body.

There has been a recent increase in teachings commonly known as functional or integrative medicine. Integrative medicine, as defined by US National Center for Complementary and Alternative Medicine (NCCAM), combines conventional medical treatments and alternative treatments for which there is some high-quality scientific evidence of safety and effectiveness. It is a concept that is now getting the attention of many academic health centers. It is important to note that integrative medicine is not synonymous with complementary and alternative medicine (CAM). It has a far larger meaning and mission, in that it calls for a return to health and healing as the focus of medicine and emphasizes the centrality of the patient-physician relationship.

In addition to providing the best conventional care, integrative medicine focuses on preventative maintenance of health by paying attention to all relative components of lifestyle, including diet, exercise, stress management, and emotional well-being. It insists on patients being active participants in healthcare, as well as on physicians viewing patients as whole persons—minds, community members, and spiritual beings—not just as physical bodies. It is a philosophy that neither rejects conventional medicine nor accepts alternative therapies uncritically, and one that uses natural, effective, and less invasive interventions whenever possible. Finally, it asks physicians to serve as guides, role models, and mentors, and not only as dispensers of therapeutic aids.

Integrative optometry follows many of these same principles. The eye maintains inherent healing abilities. For example, lysozyme in tears is a natural antibiotic. If a doctor balances the tear film through proper nutrition and flushes the eye with lubricating drops, tears themselves can fight potential infection. Research is finding that many eye conditions are actually extensions of general nutritional status, so it follows that general nutrition may improve eye conditions. Studies on nutrients and combinations of nutrients and their possible roles in eye health are ongoing.

You'll often hear that vitamins and minerals are not regulated. There are, however, regulations concerning dietary supplements, and they are enforced by the Food and Drug Administration (FDA). The Dietary Supplement Health and Education Act (DSHEA) was enacted in 1994 and defines a dietary supplement as "a product taken by mouth that contains a dietary ingredient that may include vitamins, minerals, herbs or other botanicals, amino acids and substances such as enzymes, organ tissues, glandular and metabolites." These products must have a disclaimer that says, "These statements have not been evaluated by the Food and Drug Administration. This product is not intended to diagnose, cure, prevent or treat any disease." This means that these products are considered similar to foods, not drugs. It is clear that nutrients can heal the body and alleviate illness (e.g., vitamin C for scurvy, vitamin D for rickets), but it is still the responsibility of supplement companies to manufacture their products according to cGMP (current Good Manufacturing Practices) standards and to use GRAS (Generally Recognized as Safe) ingredients. These concepts are mandated by the FDA.

FDA regulations dictate that food and dietary supplements do not need "pre-market approval," which is mandatory for drugs. Drugs, however, do not need "pre-market notification," contrary to both food and dietary supplements, which do. A pre-market submission made to the FDA must demonstrate that the device (or nutrient, in this case) to be marketed is at least as safe and effective—that is, substantially equivalent—as a legally marketed nutrient not subject to pre-market approval. Dietary supplements and drugs maintain the same requirements in the areas of labeling, GMP facility registration, and advertising. Food does not require mandatory adverse event reporting, while dietary supplements and drugs do. Since these are federal regulations, all states abide by these protocols, and the advertising issues surrounding promotion of nutrients and their benefits fall under the auspices of the Federal Trade Commission (FTC).

This handbook is divided into three parts. Part one is an overview of nutritional basics. It is meant to be used as a reference guide to the various nutrients and the ways in which they support not only the visual system but also the entire body. Part two is a listing of the common eye disorders encountered on a daily basis by practitioners. Within this listing, a brief discussion of each condition and the nutritional aspects of its treatment are offered. The charts within each section offer a number of nutritional, herbal, and homeopathic therapies that may have an influence on each disorder. Not every nutrient is required to be taken, but you will be able to see which nutrients support which ocular structures and learn the recommended dosage of each substance. Part three is a review of the nutritional approaches commonly recommended to maintain optimal health, including diet types, food choices, and homeopathic formulas.

The purpose of this book is to offer a quick and easy reference guide to use when considering integrative therapy. It is not meant to encourage you to bypass traditional Western medicine but rather to show you how to integrate other therapies with those treatments whenever appropriate. If possible, work with a doctor that maintains a referral network of nutritional professionals such as nutritionists, dietitians, chiropractors, and naturopaths. Eyecare providers should work together with these professionals—and keep the lines of communication open—for the common good of the patient. Nutritional supplements do not cure illnesses on their own, but may enhance the body's ability to fight disease. Even with medical intervention, a well-nourished body heals faster than one that is nutritionally deficient.

Nutritional supplementation is just that: a supplement to a wellness program. It is not a replacement for a good diet. Nutritional therapies provide cellular support, encouraging organs to rebalance and heal themselves. As the adage goes, "Nature heals the body but the doctor collects the fee."

PART ONE

Nutrition and Vision

Because the eyes and visual system are so integral to the body, it makes sense that they require proper nutrition to function properly over time. You might be surprised to find out that the brain and visual system use about 25 percent of the human body's nutritional intake, though they account for only about 2 percent of total body weight. It is important to identify the nutritional elements needed for the eyes and body to perform optimally.

We are what we eat. In other words, by regularly eating a moderate amount of nutrient-dense food, we may suffer far fewer diseases than by consuming empty-calorie junk food. This concept could not be simpler, yet the latest US government statistics suggest that only 11 percent of the population actually consumes five servings of fruit and vegetables a day. Just under 60 percent of the US population is now considered malnourished and clinically obese, which means moderate nutrient-dense food consumption is nowhere near the norm in this country. Interestingly, optometry can help address this nationwide health crisis by discussing the roles diet, nutrition, and portion control play in degenerative eye disease.

The following offers an overview of nutrition, including macronutrients and micronutrients. It explains how these elements of nutrition work and generally affect the body. Much of this information is akin to that which an eye care professional would learn in general physiology courses, and it is reproduced here as a handy guide for building a working knowledge of nutrition as it applies to the visual system.

DIGESTION, ABSORPTION, AND METABOLISM

Proper nutrition involves consuming foods that supply the correct nutrients in adequate amounts for optimal health. The foods eaten by humans are chemically complex and must be broken down by the body into simpler forms in order to be taken in through the intestinal wall and transported by the blood to the body's various cells. In the cells, they provide energy and building materials to maintain life. The processes that work to complete these jobs are digestion, absorption, and metabolism.

Digestion

Digestion is a series of physical and chemical processes that break down food in preparation for the absorption of its nutrients through the intestinal tract into the bloodstream. These processes take place in the digestive tract, which includes the mouth, pharynx, esophagus, stomach, small intestine, and large intestine. The active materials in the digestive juices that cause the chemical breakdown of food are known as enzymes. Enzymes are complex proteins that are capable of inducing chemical changes in other substances without being changed themselves. Each enzyme has the ability to break down a single specific substance. For example, an enzyme capable of breaking down fat cannot also break down protein or carbohydrate.

Digestion actually begins in the mouth, where large pieces of food become smaller pieces of food through the act of chewing. The salivary glands in the mouth produce saliva, a fluid that moistens the food for swallowing and contains an enzyme necessary for carbohydrate digestion. This speaks to the importance of breaking down carbohydrates quickly and thoroughly to prepare them for the digestive activity. Active chemical digestion begins in the middle portion of the stomach, where the food is mixed with gastric juices containing hydrochloric acid, water, and enzymes that deal with proteins and other substances. After one to four hours, muscle action pushes the food, now in liquid form, out of the stomach and into the small intestine. When the liquid food enters the small intestine, the pancreas secretes digestive juices, which are added to the mixture. If fats are present in the food, bile—an enzyme produced by the liver and stored in the gallbladder—is secreted. The pancreas also secretes a substance that neutralizes the digestive acids in the food, as well as additional enzymes that continue the breakdown of proteins and carbohydrates. Finally, undigested portions of the food enter the large intestine for eventual excretion. No digestive enzymes are secreted in the large intestine, and little occurs there aside from absorption of water.

Absorption

Absorption is the process by which nutrients—in the form of glucose from carbohydrates, amino acids from proteins, and fatty acids and glycerol from fats—are taken up by the intestines and passed into the bloodstream to function in cell metabolism. Absorption takes place primarily in the small intestine. The lining of the small intestine is covered with membrane protrusions known as microvilli. These microvilli contain lymph channels called lacteals and capillaries, which are the principal channels of absorption. About 60 to 70 percent of fat and fat-soluble vitamins are absorbed by lacteals into the lymphatic system and transported to the liver. The remaining nutrients are absorbed by capillaries into the bloodstream and transported to the liver.

In the liver, many different enzymes help to change the nutrient molecules into new forms for specific purposes. Unlike the earlier changes, which prepared the nutrients for absorption and transport, reactions in the liver produce the actual products needed by the cells. Some of these products are used by the liver itself, but the rest are held in storage by the liver to be released as needed into the bloodstream. From the blood, they are picked up by individual cells and put to work.

Metabolism

Metabolism is the final stage of food handling. It includes all the biochemical changes nutrients undergo from the time they are absorbed until they either become a part of the body or are excreted by it. Metabolism is the conversion of digested nutrients into building materials for living tissues or energy to meet the body's needs.

Metabolism occurs in two general phases, anabolism and catabolism, which take place simultaneously. Anabolism involves all the chemical reactions nutrients undergo in the construction or building up of body chemicals and tissues such as blood, enzymes, hormones, and glycogen. Catabolism involves all the reactions that break down various compounds and tissues to supply energy. Energy for cells is derived primarily from the metabolism of glucose, which combines with oxygen in a series of chemical reactions to form carbon dioxide, water, and cellular energy. The carbon dioxide and water are waste products, carried away from the cells by the bloodstream. Energy is also derived from the metabolism of essential fatty acids and amino acids, although the major purpose of amino-acid metabolism is to provide material for the growth, maintenance, and repair of various tissues. The waste products of the metabolism of essential fatty acids and amino acids are also carried away from the cells by the force of the bloodstream.

The process of metabolism requires that the body maintain extensive systems of enzymes to facilitate the thousands of different chemical reactions that take place and to regulate the rate at which these reactions occur. These enzymes often require the presence of specific vitamins and minerals to perform their functions. For proper growth, the body needs water, carbohydrates, proteins, and fats—called macronutrients—as well as vitamins and minerals—called micronutrients. This part of the book will describe these different nutrients and explain how they interact to supply the body—and more specifically, the eyes—with the materials required to maintain the amazing function of vision.

MACRONUTRIENTS

Macronutrients are an essential part of nutrition. They include water, carbohydrates, proteins, and fats, all of which are required for proper metabolism. Although macronutrients are critical, there are no federal guidelines regarding their intake, such as there are for vitamins and minerals. All macronutrients are required to some degree and may be found in the foods we eat. Let's review macronutrients and see how they interact with our bodies to supply the fuel for life.

Water

Water is involved in every function of the body. It helps transport nutrients and waste products in and out of cells. It is necessary for all the digestive, absorptive, circulatory, and excretory functions of the body, as well as for the body's utilization of water-soluble vitamins. It is also needed for the maintenance of proper body temperature. The human body is two-thirds water. Replenishing the body's supply of water, which is continually drained through sweating and elimination, is very important. To keep the body functioning properly, it has been widely stated that at least eight

8-ounce glasses of quality water should be ingested each day. To my knowledge, there are no actual studies that confirm this amount as absolutely necessary, but adequate hydration is always a good idea. While the body can survive without food for about five weeks, it cannot survive without water for more than five days.

Carbohydrate

Carbohydrate is the main source of blood glucose, which fuels the body and is a particularly important source of energy for the brain and red blood cells. Carbohydrates form the largest group of foods consumed by most people. This makes sense, as they are the quickest source of energy, getting converted into simple sugars and then into glucose. This glucose is then used directly to provide the body with energy or stored in the liver for future use. When a person consumes more calories than the body needs, many of the carbohydrates may also be stored as fat. Thus, when too many carbohydrates are consumed or not processed properly, excess fatty tissue accumulates.

Carbohydrates are divided into two groups: simple and complex. Complex carbohydrates include whole grains, vegetables, and legumes, which are best consumed in their natural states. These foods are low on the glycemic index (see Glycemic Index on page 131). Complex carbohydrates are made of sugars, but the sugar molecules are strung together into longer, more complex chains. Complex carbohydrates are also typically high in fiber, which lengthens digestion time. The long digestion period for these complex carbohydrates allows the body to utilize the glucose formed from their breakdown instead of storing it in fat cells.

Simple carbohydrates, sometimes called simple sugars, include fructose (fruit sugar), sucrose (a combination of glucose and fructose also known as table sugar), and lactose (milk sugar). Fruits are among the richest natural sources of simple carbohydrates. They digest easily and don't provide an excessive amount of glucose. Fruit juice, however, contains all the sugar of fruit but not the fiber. This can be a bad thing for the body. Refined carbohydrates (think white-flour foods) are not easy to digest and cause highly concentrated amounts of glucose to enter the bloodstream, which is then quickly stored in fat cells.

The standard American diet (appropriately referred to as "SAD") contains a large amount of highly concentrated, overly refined carbohydrates, which deliver more units of sugar than can be utilized by the body in a short period of time. As mentioned, this excess glucose is converted into glycogen, which is then converted into triglycerides that are stored as body fat for future use. But this "future use" rarely occurs, as most of us don't get enough exercise. The end result is the US obesity epidemic and all the health-related challenges facing today's society, including diet-related eye problems such as diabetic retinopathy and increased risk of age-related macular degeneration (AMD).

Protein

Protein is essential to growth and development. It is needed for the man-ufacture of hormones, antibodies, enzymes, and tissue, as well as to main-tain acid-alkaline balance in the body. When proteins are consumed, they are broken down into amino acids, which are the building blocks of new proteins that can be used by the body. Some amino acids are considered nonessential. This does not mean they are unnecessary, but rather that they do not have to come from diet, as they are manufactured by the body from other amino acids. The remaining amino acids are considered essen-tial, in that they are not synthesized by the body and must be obtained from diet.

Because of the importance of consuming proteins that provide all essential amino acids, dietary proteins are divided into two groups according to the amino acids they contain. Complete proteins, which con-stitute the first group, contain ample amounts of all essential amino acids. These proteins are found in meat, fish, poultry, cheese, eggs, and milk. Incomplete proteins, which constitute the second group, contain only some essential amino acids. These proteins are found in foods such as grains, legumes, and leafy green vegetables.

Although it is important to consume the full range of amino acids, both essential and nonessential, it is not necessary to get them from meat, fish, poultry, or the other complete-protein foods. It is possible to create complete proteins by combining various incomplete protein foods. This concept is called food combining. For instance, although beans and rice are both quite rich in protein, each lacks one or more essential amino acids. When you eat beans and rice together, however, or when you com-bine other protein-rich foods, you form a complete protein that is a high-quality substitute for the protein found in meat. This is a critical concept for someone who chooses a vegetarian diet. It's not wise to give up eat-ing meat without paying attention to food combining in order to attain the proper amount of protein.

Fat

Although much attention has been focused on the need to reduce the amount of fat in the average diet, the body does need some fat. During infancy and childhood, fat is necessary for normal brain growth and development. Throughout life, it provides energy and supports growth. Fat is, in fact, the most concentrated source of energy available to the body. After the age of two, however, the body requires only small amounts of fat—much less than the level provided by the typical American diet. Fat also transports fat-soluble vitamins and keeps calcium readily available to bones and teeth.

Fat is composed of building blocks called fatty acids. Fatty acids are stored in every cell membrane of the body. They ensure cellular fluidity, acting as gatekeepers for every cell, allowing vital nutrients to enter the cell, and forcing destructive free radical debris out of the cell. There are three major categories of fatty acids: saturated, monounsaturated, and polyunsaturated. Saturated fatty acids are found primarily in animal products, including dairy items such as whole milk, cream, and cheese, and fatty meats such as beef, veal, lamb, pork, and ham. The fat marbling you see in beef and pork is composed of saturated fat. Saturated fat is generally solid at room temperature. Some vegetable products—including coconut oil, palm oil, and palm kernel oil—are also high in saturated fat. The liver uses saturated fat to manufacture cholesterol, which plays a necessary part in the creation of healthy cells.

For quite some time, the public has been told that saturated fat causes heart disease and other bodily ailments, but this is not necessarily true. Clinical studies in recent years continue to show that saturated fat in moderation is healthier for the heart and vascular system than hydrogenated vegetable oil, which contains dangerous trans fats. Trans fats are produced when manufacturers add hydrogen, heat, and a metallic ion to vegetable oil in a process called hydrogenation. Hydrogenation turns liquid oil into solid fat and increases the shelf life and stability of certain foods. Partial hydrogenation is a similar process in which the action of hydrogenation is halted during the reaction so that not all the fat is converted into trans fats. A small amount of trans fats is found naturally in dairy products, meat, and other animal-based food, but this natural version of is not as harmful as the artificial type.

Trans fats may be found in vegetable shortening, margarine, crackers, cookies, snack foods, and other foods made with or fried in partially hydrogenated oil. Trans fats raise LDL cholesterol, the "bad" cholesterol that increases the risk of coronary heart disease. It is important to note, however, that excessive saturated fat may also contribute to a rise in LDL levels. The Food and Drug Administration (FDA) has now stated that it will require the elimination of trans fats from food in the United States.

Monounsaturated fat is found mostly in vegetable and nut oils such as olive, peanut, and canola. It appears to reduce LDL blood levels without affecting HDL, the "good" cholesterol, in any way. This positive impact on LDL cholesterol, however, is relatively modest. Guidelines recommend that intake of monounsaturated fat be kept between 10 and 15 percent of total caloric intake.

Polyunsaturated fat is found in the greatest abundance in corn, soybean, safflower, and sunflower oils. Certain fish oils are also high in polyunsaturated fatty acids. Unlike saturated fat, polyunsaturated fat may actually lower your total blood cholesterol level. In other words, it may also reduce beneficial HDL. For this reason, guidelines state that intake of polyunsaturated fat should not exceed 10 percent of total calories. Also important to note is the fact that these oils contain large amounts of potentially proinflammatory omega-6 fatty acids.

There has been much chatter in the press about essential fatty acids (EFAs). Much of it is misguided in regard to their effects on the eyes. The most widely discussed EFAs are the omega-3 and the omega-6 essential fatty acids. Omega-6 fatty acids are the most plentiful in our diet. They are in most everything we eat that contains fat, including meat, most seed oils, dairy products, and eggs. Omega-3 fatty acids are available in certain seed oils and most all coldwater fatty fish. A proper balance of these fatty acids is essential for good health. The daily intake recommendation of the Institute of Medicine is 4:1—four times as many omega-6 fatty acids as omega-3 fatty acids.

Docosahexaenoic acid (DHA) and arachidonic acid (ARA) are two important fatty acids. DHA, a long-chain omega-3 fatty acid, is found in tissues throughout the body. It is a major structural and functional element of all membranes in the gray matter of the brain and the retina, and is a key component of heart tissue. DHA is important for optimal brain and eye development in infants and has been shown to support brain, eye and cardiovascular health in adults. ARA, a long-chain omega-6 fatty acid, is the principal omega-6 in the brain. It is abundant in other cells throughout the body. ARA is equally important for proper brain development in infants and is a precursor to a group of hormone-like substances called eicosanoids. Eicosanoids are important in regard to immunity, blood clotting, and other vital functions of the body. Humans obtain ARA by eating foods such as meat, eggs, and milk, whereas DHA is found in a limited selection of foods such as fatty fish and organ meat. The body can also synthesize DHA from its precursor alpha-linolenic acid (ALA), but this process is inefficient. Both fatty acids occur naturally in breast milk and support the mental and visual development of infants. The health benefits of DHA extend from prenatal development into adult life.

Both omega-6 and omega-3 fatty acids can be converted into three different types of active molecules called prostaglandins (PGEs). The first type of prostaglandin, PGE1, helps reduce inflammation and inhibits blood clotting. The second, PGE2, constricts blood vessels, increases body temperature, and encourages blood clotting. The third, PGE3, plays an important anti-inflammatory role. All three of these prostaglandins are important in the maintenance of a healthful, balanced state.

Recently there has been research on another omega fatty acid: omega-7, which is found in oil derived from the fruit of sea buckthorn. Both the seed and pulp oils of this fruit are rich in tocopherols, tocotrienols, and plant sterols. In addition, sea buckthorn pulp oil contains especially high levels of carotenoids.

Due to its unique botanical and nutritional properties, and there being no reported evidence of sea buckthorn oil causing adverse reactions or negative side effects, this oil is used as a natural treatment in connection with diseases of the mucous membranes. It has also been promoted as therapy for dry eye syndrome, but studies for this application, unfortunately, are nonexistent.

EFAs and AMD

There is evidence that a diet high in omega-3 polyunsaturated fatty acids protects against early AMD. Eating oily fish at least once per week compared with less than once per week has been associated with reduced risk of AMD. Additionally, regular consumption of DHA and eicosapentaenoic acid (EPA) sourced from fish has been linked to a decrease in AMD and may help delay onset of AMD. Omega-3s may modulate metabolic processes and diminish the effects of environmental exposures that activate molecules involved in retinal diseases. These processes and exposures include oxidative stress, ischemia, chronic light exposure, inflammation, cellular signaling and aging. In one study (AREDS2), however, omega-3 fish oil failed to show a significant effect on the progression of AMD.

DHA is also a major component of retinal photoreceptor outer segment membranes. In fact, the outer segments of photoreceptor cells have some of the highest DHA content of any cell type in the body. Biochemical properties of DHA may affect photoreceptor membrane function by altering its thickness and permeability. DHA status also affects retinal cell-signaling mechanisms involved in the process of phototransduction, which converts light into electric signals. In fact, a lack of specific EFAs has been associated with a number of alterations in retinal function.

Dosage

The American Heart Association recommends eating fish at least two times per week. In particular, fatty fish are suggested, such as anchovies, bluefish, carp, catfish, halibut, herring, lake trout, mackerel, pompano, salmon, striped sea bass, tuna (albacore), and whitefish. It is also important to consume plant-derived sources of alpha-linolenic acid, such as tofu, soybeans, walnuts, flaxseeds (ground), and canola oil, although their conversion to long-chain fatty acids is not as efficient. The World Health Organization and governmental health agencies of several countries recommend consuming 0.3 to 0.5 g of combined EPA and DHA and 0.8 to 1.1 g of alpha-linolenic acid daily.

Omega-3 fatty acids are used in some infant formulas, although effective doses have not been clearly established. Ingestion of fresh fish should be limited in young children due to the presence of potentially harmful environmental contaminants in this source of omega-3 fatty acids. Except under the direction of a physician, children should not supplement with fish oil capsules. There are, however, a few "gummy" supplements now being made with children's dosage in mind. People with an allergy or hypersensitivity to fish should avoid fish oil or omega-3 fatty acid products derived from fish. People with an allergy or hypersensitivity to nuts should avoid alpha-linolenic acid products derived from the types of nuts to which they are sensitive.

The Food and Drug Administration classifies intake of up to 3 g per day of omega-3 fatty acids from fish as GRAS (Generally Regarded as Safe). Diabetic patients, however, should exercise caution due to potential (albeit unlikely) increases in blood sugar levels. People at risk of bleeding and those with high levels of LDL should also be careful and talk to their doctors before ingesting high amounts of omega-3s. Omega-3 fatty acids lower triglyceride levels but can actually increase LDL levels by a small amount, and may increase the risk of bleeding when taken with herbs and supplements that are also believed to increase the risk of bleeding. Cases of bleeding, in fact, have been reported in combination with ginkgo biloba, garlic, and saw palmetto.

Multiple human trials have reported small reductions in blood pressure with intake of omega-3 fatty acids. Reductions of 2 to 5 mmHg have been observed, and effects appear to be dose-responsive (higher doses have greater effects). DHA may have a greater effect than EPA. Caution is warranted in patients with low blood pressure and in those taking blood pressure-lowering medications. Finally, as fish (mainly large fish) may contain methylmercury, caution is warranted in connection with young children and women who are pregnant or breastfeeding.

Gastrointestinal upset is common with the use of fish oil supplements. Diarrhea may also occur, with potentially severe diarrhea at very high doses. There are also reports of increased burping, acid reflux, heartburn, indigestion, abdominal bloating, and abdominal pain. A fishy aftertaste is common, especially if the oil has gone rancid. Gastrointestinal side effects can be minimized if fish oils are taken with meals and if dosages begin low and gradually increase. Keeping the pills in the refrigerator or freezer may also reduce the incidence of digestive upset.

As fish oil supplementation over many months may cause a deficiency of vitamin E, vitamin E is added to many commercial fish oil products. This addition also reduces oxidation and spoilage. Fish liver oil contains vitamins A and D. Therefore, fish liver oil products (such as cod liver oil) may increase the risk of vitamin A or D toxicity if taken in excess. Increases in LDL by 5 to 10 percent have been observed in connection with intake of omega-3 fatty acids. Effects are dose-dependent, so low doses (half a teaspoon twice a week) are recommended.

Recommended Ratio of Macronutrients

You may now be wondering what constitutes a good dietary balance of macronutrients. Most experts agree that a good diet consists of about 2,000 calories a day. The recommended macronutrient ratio consists of about 30 percent (600 calories) fat, only 7 percent of which should be saturated fat, with the rest being mostly monounsaturated fat; 50 to 60 percent carbohydrate (1,000 to 1,200 calories), made up of mostly low-glycemic index complex carbohydrates; and 10 to 20 percent (200 to 400 calories) protein. These amounts may vary from one individual to another but are generally considered a good starting point for a healthy diet. If someone is already overweight or obese, however, a caloric reduction (under 2,000 calories a day) is warranted.

MICRONUTRIENTS—VITAMINS

Just like macronutrients, vitamins are essential to life and are therefore also considered nutrients. They are needed in such small amounts, however, that they are called micronutrients. Vitamins contribute to good health by regulating metabolism and assisting biochemical processes that release energy from digested food. Some vitamins are water-soluble, meaning they are able to be dissolved in water, while others are fat-soluble, meaning they are able to be dissolved in fat. Water-soluble vitamins must be taken into the body throughout the day, as they cannot be stored and are excreted within several hours if not used by the body. These include the B vitamins and vitamin C. Fat-soluble vitamins may be stored by the body for longer periods of time, typically in fatty tissues and the liver. These include vitamins A, D, E, and K. The body needs both the water-soluble and fat-soluble vitamins in order to function properly.

The United States developed the Dietary Reference Intake (DRI) system to refer to sufficient daily intake levels of nutrients such as vitamins and minerals. This system includes Recommended Daily Allowance (RDA) values, which refer to the nutrient amounts adequate for maintaining a baseline level of health—that is, free of disease. RDAs, however, do not promote optimal health. If you are active, under great stress, on a restricted diet, mentally or physically ill, taking medication, recovering from surgery, or a habitual smoker or drinker, you will likely need higher than normal amounts of nutrients. Women who take oral contraceptives will also require increased amounts.

The following chapter provides a list of vitamins and notes the RDA of each. Whenever applicable, it also includes a "consensus recommendation," which refers to the amount most nutritionists deem necessary for optimal health.

Vitamin A and Beta-Carotene

Of all the micronutrients important to visual function, vitamin A is probably the most recognized. Vitamin A is a fat-soluble vitamin that occurs in a variety of chemical forms. It is found as retinol in animal tissue. It is found as beta-carotene in plants, with the highest amounts present in fruits such as apricots and cantaloupes, and in vegetables such as carrots, pumpkins, sweet potatoes, spinach, squash, and broccoli. While retinol is readily absorbed by the body, beta-carotene must be broken down before it can function as a vitamin. Beta-carotene is a carotenoid, a class of compounds related to vitamin A that is converted into vitamin A in the liver.

The retina requires vitamin A to transform light energy into nerve impulses. A lack of vitamin A can cause some forms of night blindness, or nyctalopia. Since vitamin A also helps to maintain the mucous lining of various tissues, including the eye, it is important in the support of proper tear levels and prevention of dry eye syndrome. In addition, Vitamin A enhances immunity. It protects against colds, influenza, and infections of the kidneys, bladder, and lungs. It may also heal gastrointestinal ulcers, acts as an antioxidant, protects against pollution, and plays an important role in the formation of bones and teeth.

Vitamin A is primarily absorbed in the upper intestinal tract, where fat-splitting enzymes and bile salts convert carotene into a usable nutrient. The conversion of carotene into vitamin A is never 100-percent effective. Approximately one-third of the carotene in food is converted into vitamin A. Less than one-fourth of the carotene in carrots and root vegetables undergoes conversion, and about one-half of the carotene in leafy green vegetables becomes vitamin A. In addition, humans do not convert beta-carotene as readily into vitamin A as they age. Some unchanged carotene is absorbed into the circulatory system and stored in fat tissue rather than in the liver. Unabsorbed carotene is excreted.

The degree to which carotene is utilized by the body varies according to food source and food preparation method. Cooking, puréeing, or mashing of a vegetable ruptures the cell membranes, making the carotene more available for absorption. Factors interfering with the absorption of vitamin A and carotene include strenuous physical activity performed within four hours of consumption, intake of mineral oil, excessive consumption of alcohol, excessive consumption of iron, and the use of cortisone or similar medications. Diabetics have difficulty converting carotene into vitamin A. Ingesting polyunsaturated fatty acids with carotene results in rapid destruction of the carotene unless antioxidants also are present. Even cold weather can hinder the transport and metabolism of vitamin A and carotene.

Approximately 90 percent of the body's vitamin A is stored in the liver, with small amounts deposited in fat tissue, the lungs, the kidneys, and the retinas. Under stressful conditions, the body uses this reserve supply if it doesn't receive enough vitamin A from the diet. Gastrointestinal and liver disorders, infections of any kind, and any condition in which the bile duct is obstructed may limit the body's capacity to retain and use vitamin A. Factors affecting the absorption of vitamin A include the amount of the nutrient consumed, the influence of other substances present in the intestines, and the amount of the vitamin stored in the body. For these reasons, recommended dietary amounts vary.

The issue of vitamin A is a controversial topic in the eyecare profession. Vitamin A has been successfully used to treat several eye disorders, including Bitot's spots, blurred vision, true night blindness, and cataract. Therapeutic dosages of vitamin A are necessary for the treatment of dry eye syndrome and some forms of conjunctivitis. Taking large amounts of vitamin A over long periods of time, however, can be toxic to the body, mainly the liver. Research indicates that no more than 50,000 IU (International Units) per day of vitamin A may be utilized by the body except in therapeutic cases, in which up to 100,000 IU may be recommended, but only for short periods of time. Do not ingest excess vitamin A without first consulting a physician. Toxic levels of vitamin A are associated with abdominal pain, amenorrhea, enlargement of the liver and spleen, gastrointestinal disturbances, hair loss, itching, joint pain, nausea and vomiting, and cracked or scaly lips. Vitamin C may prevent the harmful effects of vitamin A toxicity. Overdose is unlikely with beta-carotene or a carotenoid complex, although an individual's skin may turn slightly yellow-orange in color due to excessive intake. The RDA of vitamin A is 3,000 IU for adult males, while the RDA for adult females is 2,300 IU. The consensus recommendations mirror these amounts. These requirements increase during periods of disease, trauma, pregnancy, and lactation. These requirements also vary for people who smoke, live in highly polluted areas, easily absorb vitamin A, or have pneumonia or nephritis.

Vitamin B Complex

B vitamins are water-soluble substances that can be cultivated from bacteria, yeasts, fungi, or molds. The known B complex vitamins are B_1 (thiamine), B_2 (riboflavin), B_3 (niacin), B_5 (pantothenic acid), B_6 (pyridoxine), B_7 (biotin), B_9 (folic acid), B_{12} (cyanocobalamin), and choline. The grouping of these water-soluble compounds under the term "B complex" is based upon their common sources, their close relationship in vegetable and animal tissues, and their functions.

B complex vitamins play an active role in providing the body with energy by converting carbohydrates into glucose, which the body burns to produce energy. They are vital in the metabolism of fats and proteins. In addition, B vitamins are necessary elements of a properly functioning nervous system and in the health of nerves. They are essential to the maintenance of muscle tone in the gastrointestinal tract, and to the health of the skin, hair, eyes, mouth, and liver.

All B vitamins are natural constituents of brewer's yeast, liver, and whole grains. Brewer's yeast, in particular, is the richest natural source of the B complex group. Another important source of B vitamins is intestinal bacteria.

Because of the water solubility of B complex vitamins, any excess is excreted rather than stored. Therefore, B vitamins must be continually replaced. All B vitamins are readily absorbed when mixed with saliva. Sulfa drugs, barbiturates, insecticides, and estrogen can create a condition in the digestive tract that can destroy B vitamins, and certain B vitamins are lost through perspiration.

The most important thing to remember is that all B vitamins should be taken together. They are so interrelated in function that a large dose of any one of them may cause a deficiency of other B vitamins. In nature, we find B complex vitamins in yeast and green vegetables, but nowhere do we find a single B vitamin isolated from the rest. The need for the B complex vitamins increases during infection and stress. Alcoholics and individuals who consume excessive amounts of carbohydrates require higher intakes of B vitamins for proper metabolism. Coffee consumption lowers levels of B vitamins. Children and pregnant women need extra B vitamins for normal growth.

B vitamins are so deficient in the American diet that almost every person in this country lacks some of them. If you are tired, irritable, nervous, depressed, or even suicidal, suspect a vitamin B deficiency. Gray hair, acne and other skin problems, poor appetite, insomnia, neuritis, anemia, constipation, and a high cholesterol level are also indicators of vitamin B deficiency. One reason there is such a great vitamin B deficiency in the American population is that we eat so much processed food, which loses B vitamins during manufacturing. Another reason for the widespread deficiency is the high amount of sugar people consume. Sugar and alcohol destroy B complex vitamins.

Massive doses of B complex vitamins have been used to treat polio, improve the condition of hypersensitive children who fail to respond favorably to medications such as Ritalin, and battle cases of shingles. Nervous individuals and persons working under tension can greatly benefit from taking larger than normal doses of B vitamins. B vitamins may also treat beriberi (caused by vitamin B_1 deficiency), pellagra (caused by a shortage of vitamin B_3, specifically nicotinic acid), constipation, burning feet, tender gums, eyelid twitching, diplopia, fatigue, lack of appetite, skin disorders, cracks at the corners of the mouth, anemia, and dry eye.

Vitamin B_1 (Thiamine)

Vitamin B_1, also known as thiamine, combines with pyruvic acid to form a coenzyme necessary to convert carbohydrate into glucose, which is then oxidized by the body to produce energy. Thiamine is vulnerable to heat, air, and water in cooking. It is a component of the germ and bran of wheat, the husk of rice, and that portion of all grains which is commercially milled away to give the grain a lighter color and finer texture. Thiamine enhances circulation, assists in the formation of blood, and aids in the production of hydrochloric acid. Thiamine also optimizes cognitive activity and brain function. It has a positive effect on energy, growth, appetite, and learning capacity, and is needed for muscle tone in the intestines, stomach, and heart. It also acts as an antioxidant, protecting the body from the degenerative effects of aging, alcohol consumption, and smoking.

Thiamine deficiency can lead to optic neuritis, as well as to impairment of the central nervous system. The first signs of thiamine deficiency include fatigue, loss of appetite, irritability, and emotional instability. If the deficiency is not addressed, confusion and loss of memory appear, followed closely by gastric distress, abdominal pain, and constipation.

The RDA of thiamine is 1.2 milligrams (mg) for adult men and 1.1 mg for adult women (1.4 mg for pregnant or lactating women). The consensus recommendation is 25 mg per day. The need for thiamine increases during severe diarrhea, fever, stress, and surgery. Thiamine has no known toxic side effects. The richest food sources of thiamine are brown rice, egg yolks, fish, legumes, liver, pork, poultry, rice bran, wheat germ, and whole grains. Many herbs also contain thiamine.

Vitamin B_2 (Riboflavin)

Vitamin B_2, also known as riboflavin, is a vitamin that occurs naturally in the same foods containing the other B vitamins. Riboflavin is stable to heat, oxidation, and acid, but disintegrates in the presence of alkalis or light, especially UV light.

To support mitochondrial energy production, riboflavin functions as part of a group of enzymes involved in the breakdown and utilization of carbohydrate, fat, and protein. It is necessary for cell respiration because it works with enzymes in the utilization of cell oxygen. It is required for red blood cell formation and respiration, antibody production, growth, and reproduction. It's also solely responsible for the fluorescent-yellow color in urine of people who supplement with high-dose B vitamins. It also helps in the prevention of many types of eye disorders, including conjunctival infection, itching or burning eyes, cataract, and photophobia. Low levels of vitamin B_2 have been linked to excessive ingrowth of blood vessels into the cornea.

Increased occurance of age-related cataract has been shown in those who are deficient in vitamin B_2. One Australian study of both men and women suggested the incident of age-related cataract was half as likely in those with the highest riboflavin intake as in those in the lowest riboflavin intake.

Riboflavin drops and UV light exposure are now used in the process of corneal cross-linking to treat patients with progressive keratoconus and other corneal dystrophies. Riboflavin has also been used in a number of studies to address the impaired mitochondrial oxygen metabolism in the brain that has been linked to chronic migraine headaches. Although the findings are preliminary, data suggests that riboflavin supplementation might lead to migraine prevention. It is necessary for good vision and healthy skin, nails, and hair.

Vitamin B_2 deficiency is rarely found in isolation and occurs frequently in combination with deficiencies of other water-soluble vitamins. Symptoms can include, sore throat, redness and swelling of the lining of the mouth and throat, cracks or sores on the outside of the lips and corners of the mouth, inflammation and redness of the tongue, and moist, scaly skin, particularly affecting the scrotum or labia majora and the nasolabial folds. This deficiency can result from poor dietary habits, alcoholism, or prolonged dietary restriction.

The RDA of riboflavin is 1.3 mg for adult males and 1.2 mg for adult females (1.6 mg for pregnant or lactating women). The consensus recommendation is 10 mg per day. According to the Food & Nutrition Board at the Institute of Medicine, no toxic or adverse effects of high supplemental riboflavin intake in humans are known. Excessive amounts of this vitamin, however, can make a person extremely sensitive to light, and prolonged ingestion of large doses of any one of the B complex vitamins may result in high urinary losses of other B vitamins. Therefore, it is important to take a complete B complex supplement when taking any single B vitamin.

Milk, cheese, eggs, almonds, salmon, chicken, beef, broccoli, asparagus, spinach, and fortified breads are the main food sources of riboflavin.

Vitamin B₃ (Niacin)

Niacin (nicotinic acid) is another member of the B complex family of vitamins and is also water-soluble. It is more stable than both thiamine and riboflavin, and is remarkably resistant to heat, light, air, acids, and alkalis. Niacin assists enzymes in the breakdown and utilization of proteins, fats, and carbohydrates. It is effective at improving circulation and increasing HDL cholesterol levels. It is vital to the proper functioning of the nervous system, and crucial to the formation and maintenance of healthy tongue and digestive system tissues, as well as skin.

Relatively small amounts of pure niacin are present in most foods. The niacin equivalent listed in dietary tables refers either to pure niacin or to tryptophan, an amino acid that can be converted into niacin by the body. Lean meats, poultry, fish, and peanuts are rich sources of both niacin and tryptophan, as are such dietary supplements as brewer's yeast, wheat germ, and desiccated liver. Niacin is difficult to obtain except from these foods. Excessive consumption of sugar and starches depletes the body's supply of niacin, as does taking certain antibiotics. There are many symptoms of niacin deficiency. In the early stages, they include muscular weakness, general fatigue, loss of appetite, indigestion, and various skin eruptions. Niacin deficiency may also cause bad breath, small ulcers, canker sores, insomnia, irritability, nausea, vomiting, headaches, tender gums, strain, tension, and deep depression.

The RDA of niacin is 16 mg for males and 14 mg for females (18 mg for pregnant women, 17 mg for lactating women). The consensus recommendation is 50 mg per day. There have been no toxic side effects reported for niacin, but taking extremely large doses can cause tingling and itching sensations, intense flushing of the skin, and throbbing of the head. It may also lead to a condition called cystoid maculopathy, which is reversible when large doses are stopped. The maximum suggested dose for treatment of HDL cholesterol is 2,000 mg per day. If used for this reason, the patient should start with a daily dose of 500 mg at bedtime (with some food in the stomach) for about a month, gradually adding another pill of 500 mg each month while rechecking HDL levels. Most times, this amount will be adequate for cholesterol control. Most people will sleep through the skin flush. The "non-flush" form of niacin (niacinamide) is not an effective means of HDL modification.

Vitamin B₅ (Pantothenic Acid)

Pantothenic acid, also known as vitamin B₅, is required for the conversion of carbohydrates, fats, and proteins into usable energy for the body. It is necessary for steroid metabolism, and the synthesis of red blood cells, fatty acids, and cholesterol. It is the precursor of coenzyme A (CoA), which is necessary for mitochondrial ATP energy production.

Pantothenic acid deficiency results in diminished adrenal gland function. A variety of metabolic problems will also manifest themselves. Fatigue, depression, and digestive problems are common symptoms. There might also be loss of nerve function, as well as problems with blood sugar metabolism—hypoglycemia being the most typical. Pantothenic acid deficiency can reduce immune system response, increasing the risk of infection.

Small quantities of pantothenic acid are found in most foods. The major food source of pantothenic acid is meat. Whole grains are another good source of the vitamin, but milling often removes much of the pantothenic acid, as it is found in the outer layers of whole grains. Vegetables such as broccoli and avocados have an abundance of the acid. It is also apparent in rice, wheat bran, alfalfa, peanut meal, molasses, yeast, and condensed fish solutions.

The RDA of vitamin B₅ is 5 mg for adults (6 mg for pregnant women, 7 mg for lactating women). The consensus recommendation is 50 mg per day.

Vitamin B₆ (Pyridoxine)

Vitamin B₆ consists of three related compounds—pyridoxine, pyridoxinal, and pyridoxamine. It is required for the proper absorption of vitamin B₁₂, and for the production of hydrochloric acid and magnesium. Pyridoxine, along with the other B vitamins, plays an important role as a coenzyme in the breakdown and utilization of carbohydrates, fats, and proteins. It is required for the production of antibodies and red blood cells. In addition, it facilitates the release of glycogen for energy from the liver and muscles. Vitamin B_6 helps to maintain the balance between sodium and potassium, which regulate body fluids and promote the normal functioning of the nervous and musculoskeletal systems. The best sources of vitamin B_6 are meat and whole grains, specifically desiccated liver and brewer's yeast.

The RDA of vitamin B_6 is 1.3 mg, which increases to 1.7 mg after the age of fifty. The need for vitamin B_6 almost doubles during pregnancy (1.9 mg per day) and lactation (2 mg per day). The consensus recommendation is 50 mg.

Approximately 10 percent of the US population consumes less than half the RDA of B_6. Deficiency may cause loss of hair, water retention during pregnancy, cracks around the mouth and eyes, numbness and cramps in the arms and legs, slow learning, visual disturbances, neuritis, arthritis, heart disorders, and increased urination.

Vitamin B₇ (Biotin)

Vitamin B_7, also known as biotin or vitamin H, is used in cell growth, the production of fatty acids, and the metabolism of fats and proteins. It is required for healthy hair, skin, sweat glands, nerve tissue, and bone marrow, and assists with muscle pain. It also helps in the transfer of carbon dioxide and the maintenance of a steady blood sugar level.

Although biotin deficiency is very rare, it can happen, and may result in dry skin, fatigue, loss of appetite, nausea and vomiting, mental depression, tongue inflammation, and high cholesterol. Biotin deficiency may also cause a depletion of the amino acid glycine in the body.

The RDA of biotin is 30 micrograms (mcg) for adults (35 mcg for lactating women), while the consensus recommendation is 1,000 mcg.

Vitamin B₉ (Folic Acid)

Folic acid functions as a coenzyme together with vitamins B_{12} and C in the breakdown and utilization of proteins. Folic acid performs its basic role as a carbon carrier in the formation of heme, the iron-containing protein found in hemoglobin, which is required in the formation of red blood cells. It also is needed in the creation of nucleic acid, which is essential to the process of growth and reproduction of all cells. Folic acid also increases the appetite and stimulates production of hydrochloric acid, which helps to prevent intestinal parasites and food poisoning. In addition, it supports liver function. Folic acid is easily destroyed by high temperature, exposure to light, and being left at room temperature for long periods of time. The best sources of folic acid are green leafy vegetables, liver, and brewer's yeast.

Folic acid is absorbed in the gastrointestinal tract by active transport and diffusion and stored primarily in the liver. Sulfa drugs may interfere with intestinal bacteria that manufacture folic acid.

Unmethylated folic acid is a synthetic form of folate typically found in nutritional supplements. Synthetic folic acid is metabolized by the body into levomefolic acid, which is the active form of folic acid. Approximately 10 percent of the general population lack the enzymes needed to receive any benefit from folic acid supplementation. Another 40 percent appear to convert only a limited amount of folic acid into levomefolic acid. They cannot fully process supplemental folic acid at RDA or higher dosages. Therefore, look for high quality nutritional supplements that use the methylated form of folate.

A study published in 2009 reported that use of a nutritional supplement containing folic acid, pyridoxine, and cyanocobalamin decreased the risk of developing age-related macular degeneration by 34.7 percent.

Almost any interference with the metabolism of folic acid in a fetus encourages deformities such as cleft pallet, brain damage, spina bifida, slow development, and poor learning ability in the child. In addition, deficiency of folic acid leads to toxemia, premature birth, afterbirth hemorrhaging, and megaloblastic anemia in both mother and child. Therefore, most, if not all, prenatal vitamins contain folic acid.

The recommended daily allowance of folic acid is 400 mcg for adults (600 mcg for pregnant women, 500 mcg for lactating women). The consensus recommendation is 1 mg per day. Stress and disease increase the body's need for folic acid, as does the consumption of alcohol. There is no known toxicity level of this vitamin, although excessive intake of folic acid can mask a vitamin B_{12} deficiency. A prescription is required for doses higher than 400 mcg per tablet.

Vitamin B_{12} (Cyanocobalamin)

Vitamin B_{12} is unique in that it is the first cobalt-containing substance found to be required for longevity. In addition, it is the only vitamin that contains essential mineral elements. Vitamin B_{12} cannot be made synthetically, but must be grown, like penicillin, in bacteria or molds. One of the only foods in which B_{12} occurs naturally in substantial amounts is animal protein. Therefore, vegetarians are frequently low in vitamin B_{12}. As stated, high blood levels of folic acid can mask a vitamin B_{12} deficiency.

Liver is the best source of B_{12}, while kidneys, meat, fish, and dairy products are other good sources.

As with all B vitamins, vitamin B_{12} is necessary for the normal metabolism of nerve tissue, and is involved in protein, fat, and carbohydrate metabolism. Vitamin B_{12} is taken into the mitochondria and plays an important role in amino acid metabolism. Vitamin B_{12} also helps iron to function better in the body, and aids folic acid in the synthesis of choline.

A B_{12} deficiency has been shown to affect 10 to 15 percent of individuals over the age of sixty in the United States. Patients with B_{12} deficiency may exhibit megaloblastic anemia and often hyperhomocysteinemia, which has been associated with increasing the risk of dry macular degeneration progressing to wet macular degeneration. The symptoms of a vitamin B_{12} deficiency may take five to six years to appear. Deficiency of this nutrient is usually due to a lack of the intrinsic factor, a glycoprotein necessary for absorption of this vitamin. Deficiency begins with changes in the nervous system such as soreness and weakness in the legs and arms, diminished reflex response and sensory perception, difficulty walking and speaking, and jerking of the limbs.

The condition of tobacco amblyopia, which includes symptoms such as blackouts, headaches, and hyperopia, has been improved with injections of vitamin B_{12}, whether or not the patient stopped smoking. No cases of vitamin B_{12} toxicity have ever been reported. Findings support the hypothesis that cyanocobalamin is an endogenous superoxide scavenger where depletion may result in optic neuropathy.

The RDA of vitamin B_{12} is 2.4 mcg for adults (2.6 mcg for pregnant women, 2.8 mcg for lactating women), while the consensus recommendation is 1 mg per day.

Choline

Choline is a water-soluble essential nutrient that is typically grouped together with the B complex vitamins. It is present in all living cells, and is widely distributed in animal and plant tissues. Rich dietary sources of choline include egg yolk, liver, brewer's yeast, and wheat germ.

Choline appears to be associated primarily with the treatment of fat and cholesterol in the body. It prevents fat from accumulating in the liver and facilitates its movement into cells. In the liver, choline combines with fatty acids and phosphoric acid to form lecithin. It is essential to the health of the liver and kidneys. Choline also plays an important role in the transmission of nerve impulses, as it promotes healthy myelin sheaths. Choline helps to regulate and improve liver and gallbladder function, and aids in the prevention of gallstones.

The RDA of choline is 550 mg for males and 425 mg for females (450 mg for pregnant women, 550 mg for lactating women), while the consensus recommendation is 550 mg per day.

Vitamin C

Vitamin C, also known as ascorbic acid, is another water-soluble nutrient. Although fairly stable in acidic solutions, it is normally the least stable of the vitamins and is very sensitive to oxygen. Its potency can be lost through exposure to light, heat, or air, all of which stimulate the activity of oxidative enzymes.

The primary function of vitamin C is to maintain the body's collagen, a protein necessary in the formation of the sclera—also known as the white of the eye. One school of thought regarding the effect of vitamin C on the development of myopia is that since the vitamin fortifies the sclera, a lack of vitamin C over an extended period of time—especially during growth years—weakens the scleral structure and allows the pressure inside the eye to expand the length of the eye, leading to myopia.

Vitamin C plays a role in the healing of wounds and burns because it facilitates formation of connective tissue in scars. Vitamin C also aids in the creation of red blood cells and the prevention of hemorrhaging. In addition, vitamin C fights bacterial infections and reduces the effects of some allergens. For these reasons, vitamin C is frequently promoted for the prevention and treatment of the common cold.

Vitamin C is present in most fresh fruits and vegetables. Natural vitamin C dietary supplements are prepared from sources such as rose hips, acerola cherries, green peppers, and citrus fruits. The level of ascorbic acid in the blood reaches a maximum about two to three hours after the ingestion of a moderate quantity of the nutrient, and then decreases as the vitamin is eliminated in the urine and through perspiration. Most vitamin C leaves the body within three to four hours.

Because vitamin C is considered a "stress vitamin," it is used up even more rapidly under stressful conditions. Humans, apes, and guinea pigs are the only animals that must obtain vitamin C from their food because they are unable to meet their biological needs through synthesis alone. Ascorbic acid is readily absorbed from the gastrointestinal tract into the bloodstream. Two factors that influence its absorption are the manner in which the vitamin is administered and the presence of other substances in the intestinal tract. The normal human body, when fully saturated, contains about 5,000 mg of vitamin C.

The aqueous humor of the eye maintains a vitamin C level approximately twenty-six times higher than that of blood plasma. This is considered significant in the nutrition of the lens, which depends on the aqueous fluid for its nourishment. It stands to reason that your level of vitamin C should be upheld or increased with age in an attempt to maintain a clear and healthy lens.

The RDA of vitamin C is 90 mg for adult males and 75 mg for adult females (85 mg for pregnant women, 120 mg for lactating women). The consensus recommendation is 500 mg. Dr. Linus Pauling, however, suggested 2,300 to 9,000 mg as the optimal daily intake of vitamin C for most adults. This wide range takes into account differences in weight, activity levels, metabolism, ailments, and age. Toxicity symptoms usually do not occur with high intakes of vitamin C because the body simply discharges whatever it cannot use. A daily intake of 5,000 mg to 15,000 mg, however, may cause side effects in some people. Typical toxicity symptoms of vitamin C include a slight burning sensation during urination, loose bowels, and skin rashes.

The body's ability to absorb vitamin C is reduced by smoking, stress, high fever, prolonged intake of antibiotics or cortisone, inhalation of petroleum fumes, and ingestion of aspirin or other painkillers. Baking soda destroys vitamin C, as does cooking with copper utensils. Signs of deficiency include shortness of breath, impaired digestion, poor lactation, bleeding gums, weakened tooth enamel or dentine, tendency to bruise, swollen or painful joints, nosebleeds, anemia, lowered resistance to infection, and slow healing of wounds. Severe deficiency results in scurvy.

Vitamin D

Vitamin D is a fat-soluble vitamin that can be acquired both from food and through exposure to sunlight. It is known as the "sunshine vitamin" because the sun's UV rays activate a form of cholesterol present in the skin, converting this substance into vitamin D. Although vitamin D is commonly called a vitamin, it is not, in the true sense, an essential dietary vitamin, as it can be synthesized in adequate amounts by any mammal exposed to sunlight. Nevertheless, vitamin D fits within the definition of vitamin, as it is an organic compound required as a vital nutrient in tiny amounts by an organism.

There are two forms of vitamin D. Vitamin D_2 (ergocaliferol) may be found in certain vegetables, while D_3 (cholecalciferol) may be found in some animals. D_3 is the more bioavailable form, being more effective than D_2 by about 70 percent. Oftentimes, physicians will recommend vitamin D_2 at a dosage of 50,000 IU daily for about a week, but levels will fall again quickly if such intake of vitamin D is not maintained. Vitamin D_3 can be absorbed more easily, and so is more effective at moving serum levels into the normal range.

Vitamin D aids in the absorption of calcium from the intestinal tract, and in the breakdown and assimilation of phosphorus, which is required for bone formation. In the mucous membranes, it helps in the synthesis of enzymes involved in the active transport of available calcium. Vitamin D is necessary for normal growth in children, promoting proper calcification of bones and teeth. Adults may also benefit from supplemental vitamin D, as most of them spend a majority of their days indoors. It is valuable in the maintenance of a stable nervous system, normal heart action, and normal blood clotting, as all these functions are related to the body's supply and utilization of calcium and phosphorus.

Vitamin D is best utilized by the body when taken with vitamin A. Fish liver oil (such as cod liver oil) in moderate amounts is the best natural source of vitamins A and D, although most of the body's vitamin D needs can be met by sufficient exposure to sunlight (fifteen to twenty minutes a day of summer sun exposure). The sun's action on the skin, however, may be inhibited by such factors as air pollution, clouds, window glass, and clothing. The RDA of vitamin D is set at 600 IU for adults, increasing to 800 IU for adults seventy-one years of age or older. The consensus recommendation ranges from 2,000 IU to 5,000 IU per day. The vast majority of authorities consider 2,000 IU per day a safe and effective dosage.

Being a fat-soluble vitamin means that vitamin D may be stored in the body. Excessive blood levels of this vitamin often create a rise in blood levels of calcium and phosphorus, and excessive excretion of calcium in the urine. This leads to calcification of soft tissue and the walls of blood vessels and kidney tubules, a condition known as hypercalcemia. The symptoms of an acute overdose are increased frequency of urination, loss of appetite, nausea, vomiting, diarrhea, muscular weakness, dizziness, weariness, and calcification of the soft tissues of the heart, blood vessels, and lungs. These symptoms disappear within a few days of discontinuation of vitamin D supplementation.

It is widely recognized that most adults are deficient in vitamin D, especially those individuals in extreme northern and southern latitudes, and, in particular, African Americans. A deficiency of vitamin D leads to inadequate absorption of calcium from the intestinal tract and retention of phosphorus in the kidneys. The inability of soft bones to withstand the stress of the body's weight results in skeletal malformations. Rickets, a bone disorder in children, is a direct result of vitamin D deficiency. Adult rickets, called osteomalacia, may also occur. Research suggests that vitamin D deficiency might even be a cause of myopia. An imbalance between this vitamin and calcium is likely at the root of this disorder. Other possible ocular effects include conditions such as keratoconus, conjunctivitis, cataract, and arteriosclerosis.

Vitamin E

Vitamin E refers to a group of eight fat-soluble compounds that include both tocopherols and tocotrienols. These eight forms are divided into two groups: four tocopherols and four tocotrienols. They are identified by the prefixes alpha, beta, gamma, and delta, with alpha-tocopherol being the most common in the North American diet. As an antioxidant that helps to stop the production of reactive oxygen species formed when fat undergoes oxidation, alpha-tocopherol is the most potent and has the greatest nutritional value of the group. Tocopherols occur in the highest concentrations in cold-pressed vegetable oils, whole raw seeds and nuts, and soybeans. Historically, wheat germ oil was the first source from which vitamin E was obtained.

Current science is revealing an increasingly important role for tocotrienols. A very small percentage of papers on vitamin E discuss tocotrienols, but the research is growing. Numerous recent studies have demonstrated that tocotrienols possess antioxidant, antichlosterolemic, anti-atherosclerotic, anticancer, antitumor, antihypertensive, immuno-modulatory, and neuroprotective properties. Some studies have suggested that tocotrienols have specialized roles in protecting neurons from damage and reducing cholesterol through their ability to inhibit the activity of enzyme HMG-CoA reductase (similar to the actions of statin drugs). Oral consumption of tocotrienols is also thought to protect against stroke-associated brain damage.

Vitamin E plays an essential role in the cellular respiration of muscles, especially cardiac and skeletal muscles. It makes it possible for these muscles and their nerves to function with less oxygen, thereby increasing their endurance and stamina. It also causes vasodilation, permitting a fuller flow of blood to the heart and other organs. It works to treat and prevent heart disease and can disintegrate arterial blood clots. Vitamin E is beneficial to persons with atherosclerosis if used as a therapy before irreparable damage occurs. It relieves pain in the extremities, speeds up blood flow, and reduces clotting tendencies.

In addition, vitamin E helps to counteract premature aging of the skin. It is useful to apply vitamin E to the skin while also taking it orally, as it replaces cells on the epidermal layer of the skin. Vitamin E also works against the slowdown of metabolic processes during aging.

Vitamin E therapy has been suggested as beneficial in regard to a number of other conditions, including bursitis, gout, arthritis, varicose veins, phlebitis, nephritis, and even headache. It is effective against the formation of elevated scar tissue on the surface of the body and within the body. In ointment form, it is used on burns to promote healing and to lessen the formation of scars. As a diuretic, vitamin E helps to lower elevated blood pressure. It also protects against the damaging effects of many environmental poisons in the air, water, and food.

There are several substances that interfere with, or even cause a depletion of, vitamin E. For example, when iron, especially its inorganic form, and vitamin E are administered together, absorption of each is impaired. Chlorine in drinking water, ferric chloride, rancid fat, and inorganic iron compounds destroy vitamin E in the body. Mineral oil used as a laxative depletes vitamin E. Large amounts of polyunsaturated fat or oil in the diet increase the oxidation rate of vitamin E. Thus, the more unsaturated fat or oil is consumed, the more vitamin E is necessary.

The first sign of a vitamin E deficiency is red blood cells rupturing, which is the result of the cells' increased fragility. Too little vitamin E could result in weakened membrane stability and a reduction in collagen production. A tendency towards muscular wasting or abnormal fat deposits in muscles, as well as an increased demand for oxygen may also occur. Essential fatty acids may become altered so that blood cells break down and hemoglobin formation is impaired. In addition, the body's ability to utilize several amino acids is impaired by vitamin E deficiency, as is the level of function of the pituitary and adrenal glands. Iron absorption and hemoglobin formation may also be affected. A severe deficiency can cause damage to the kidneys and liver. A prolonged deficiency of vitamin E can cause faulty absorption of fat and fat-soluble vitamins.

The RDA of vitamin E (natural alpha-tocopherol) is 22 IU for adults, including pregnant women (28 IU for lactating females). The consensus recommendation is 200 IU per day. Researchers estimate that over 80 percent of Americans do not get even the minimal required amount of vitamin E from their diets. According to Dr. Barrie Tan, distinguished researcher of Vitamin E, "Vitamin E deficiency could make us more prone to atherosclerosis or diseases that involve an enhanced production of oxygen radicals. Renegade radical molecules can rampage throughout cells, destroying lipids, proteins, and DNA. By disarming oxygen radicals, vitamin E may act as an insurance policy against oxidative stress."

Vitamin K

There are three main K vitamins. K_1 and K_2 are fat-soluble nutrients that can be manufactured in the intestinal tract. Vitamin K_3 is produced synthetically for the treatment of patients who are unable to utilize naturally occurring vitamin K due to a lack of bile.

If yogurt or fermented milk such as kefir is included in the diet, the body may be able to manufacture sufficient amounts of vitamin K. Unsaturated fatty acids and a low-carbohydrate diet increase the amounts of vitamin K produced in the intestine.

Vitamin K is absorbed in the upper intestinal tract with the aid of bile or bile salts. It is then transported to the liver where it forms pro-thrombin, a chemical necessary for blood clotting, and several related proteins. Vitamin K is also involved in phosphorylation, in which phosphate is combined with glucose and passed through cell membranes to be converted into glycogen. It is also vital for normal liver function and is an important factor in longevity. Vitamin K helps to keep calcium in bones and prevents calcium from accumulating in arteries—an important consideration, since most plaque is made of calcium.

Vitamin K is stored in very small amounts, and considerable quantities are excreted after administration of therapeutic doses. Natural sources include kelp, alfalfa, leafy greens, and green vegetables. Cow's milk, yogurt, egg yolk, blackstrap molasses, safflower oil, fish liver oil, and other polyunsaturated oils are also good sources. The most dependable supply is intestinal bacteria. Frozen foods, rancid fats, radiation, x-rays, aspirin, and industrial air pollution all destroy vitamin K. Excessive use of antibiotics can destroy intestinal flora. Ingestion of mineral oil will cause rapid excretion of vitamin K.

The RDA of vitamin K is 120 mcg for adult males and 90 mcg for adult females. The consensus recommendation is 500 mcg per day.

MICRONUTRIENTS—MINERALS

Minerals are micronutrients that exist in the body and in food, in organic and inorganic combinations. Approximately sixteen minerals are essential to proper human nutrition, and almost as many play significant roles in ocular health. Although minerals make up only 4 to 5 percent of the human body's weight, they are vital to overall mental and physical well-being. All tissues and internal fluids of living things contain varying quantities of minerals. Minerals are constituents of bones, teeth, soft tissue, muscle, blood, and nerve cells. They are important in maintaining physiological processes, strengthening skeletal structure, and preserving the vigor of the heart, brain, and all muscle and nerve systems.

It is important to note that the actions of all minerals within the body are interrelated; no one mineral functions without affecting others. In addition, physical and emotional stress can cause a strain on the body's mineral supply. A mineral deficiency often results in illness, which may be corrected by adding the missing mineral to the diet.

Boron

Although boron is not considered an essential nutrient, it is a mineral known to maintain healthy hormone levels. Through hormones, boron may play a role in ocular health. Women who develop early menopause or undergo hysterectomy have an elevated chance of developing age-related macular degeneration later in life. The reason for this may be two-fold. First, estrogen raises HDL, which transports carotenoids lutein and zeaxanthin to the eye. Secondly, estrogen helps to maintain levels of hyaluronic acid, without which retinal cells lose their support and may suffer metabolically. Therefore, if estrogen levels are too low, then eye problems may arise. Additionally, hormone levels can affect tear levels.

A rare form of corneal dystrophy known as congenital endothelial dystrophy type 2 is linked to mutations in the *SLC4A11* gene and plays a role in the intracellular concentration of boron.

While boron has no official RDA, I recommend an intake of approximately 2 mg per day for healthy adults.

Calcium

Calcium is the most abundant mineral in the body. As you may already know, most of the calcium in the body is deposited in the bones and teeth, with the remainder found in soft tissue. To function properly calcium must be accompanied by magnesium, phosphorus, and vitamins A, C, and D. Calcium helps to promote healthy blood, eases insomnia, and aids in the regulation of the heartbeat. Along with magnesium, calcium is very important to cardiovascular health. It assists in the process of blood clotting and helps to prevent the accumulation of too much acid or alkali in the blood. It also plays a part in muscle growth, muscle contraction, and nerve transmission. Calcium aids in the body's utilization of iron, helps to activate several enzymes, and plays a role in the passage of nutrients through cell walls.

The body absorbs calcium quite poorly, with only 20 to 30 percent of ingested calcium actually being absorbed. When a higher level of calcium is required, however, the body tends to take it in more effectively. Absorption ability also increases during periods of rapid growth. Calcium usage depends upon the presence of adequate amounts of vitamin D, which works with the parathyroid hormone to regulate the amount of calcium in the blood. Phosphorus is needed in at least the same amount as calcium. Vitamins A and C are also necessary for calcium absorption. Fat consumed in moderate amounts also facilitates absorption, as does a high intake of protein.

Certain substances inhibit calcium absorption. When excessive amounts of fat combine with calcium, the result is an insoluble compound that cannot be used. The combination of calcium and oxalic acid—which is found in foods such as chocolate, spinach, and rhubarb—creates another insoluble compound, which may form into stones in the kidney or gallbladder. Other interfering factors are lack of exercise, excessive stress, and too rapid a flow of food through the intestinal tract.

One of the first signs of calcium deficiency is a nervous affliction called tetany, which is characterized by muscle cramps, numbness, tingling in the arms and hands, and possibly a twitching of the eyelids. Calcium deficiency can result in bone malformation, causing rickets in children and osteomalacia in adults. Another ailment that results from calcium deficiency is osteoporosis, which occurs when calcium is withdrawn from bones, as well as from other areas of the body, faster than it is deposited.

There is a possibility of "over-calcification" with the ingestion of excessive amounts of calcium over a long period of time. This condition can lead to kidney stones, mitral valve disease, and calcification of the small and large blood vessels (including those of the eyes). It is important to note that most plaques attributed to excess cholesterol are actually comprised of more calcium (over 50 percent) than cholesterol (3 percent). The most common form of calcium likely to contribute to this issue is alkaline calcium from cheap supplements. Unfortunately, the majority of calcium supplements contain coral, dolomite, or eggshell that has been ground up. These sources are not only very difficult to absorb but also, due to their highly alkaline pH levels, potentially problematic to the body's natural state of balance.

Calcium supplements are safe, providing that patients take a full-spectrum supplement with the right form of acidified calcium together with all the cofactors for enhanced uptake and absorption. A good calcium supplement should contain chelated calcium and magnesium. It should also contain the absorption cofactors manganese, boron, copper, zinc, and strontium. Lastly, patients should take these supplements with meals. If they do so, proper calcium supplementation will continue to provide the many health benefits that have been shown in hundreds of studies over the last few decades.

The RDA of calcium is 1,000 mg for adults up to fifty years of age, and 1,200 mg for those fifty-one or older. In a standard multivitamin, only 100 mg is generally provided. Of course, if you are aiming for the RDA, more is required. A separate supplement can bridge the gap.

Chromium

Chromium is an essential mineral that stimulates the activity of enzymes involved in the metabolism of glucose for energy and the synthesis of fatty acids and cholesterol. It also appears to increase the effectiveness of insulin, thereby facilitating the transport of glucose into cells. In the blood, it competes with iron in the transport of protein. Chromium may also be involved in the synthesis of protein through its binding action with RNA molecules.

Sources of chromium include clams, whole grain cereals, and meat. Fruit and vegetables contain trace amounts. Brewer's yeast provides a dependable supply without the problem of high-carbohydrate intake or high cholesterol levels. The body retains only about 3 percent of dietary chromium, and the amount stored by the body decreases with age.

A chromium deficiency may upset the function of insulin and result in depressed growth rates and severe glucose intolerance in diabetics. It is also believed that the interaction of chromium and insulin is not limited to glucose metabolism but also affects amino acid metabolism. As well, a deficiency may contribute to atherosclerosis, as chromium may inhibit the formation of aortic plaques. Chromium deficiency has also been shown to be a factor in the development of myopia.

The RDA of chromium is 35 mcg for adult males up to age fifty and 25 mcg for adult females up to age fifty. These amounts each drop by 5 mcg for adults fifty-one and over. Pregnant women are advised to take 30 mcg per day, while lactating women should take 45 mcg. The consensus recommendation is 200 mcg per day.

Copper

Copper is a trace mineral, which means it is essential for good health but only a tiny amount is needed. When excess copper accumulates it is stored in the eyes, brain, kidneys, and liver. Excess copper collecting in the liver causes cirrhosis of the liver, which is a serious, life-threatening condition.

Wilson's disease is a treatable hereditary disorder in which the body retains too much copper. As copper is found in different amounts in a wide variety of foods, dietary restriction alone is usually not enough to control Wilson's disease, though it is helpful to avoid copper-rich foods as much as possible if you suffer from this affliction. Some of the foods rich in copper are liver, oysters, sesame seeds, cocoa powder, nuts, calamari, and sunflower seeds.

Over-consumption of copper will lead to cramps, diarrhea, and vomiting in the short term, and may lead to depression, schizophrenia, hypertension, senility, and insomnia in the long term. The stomach needs to be acidic in order to absorb copper and thus antacids interfere with the absorption of copper, as do milk and egg proteins.

A link between copper and iron metabolism has been well established. Copper deficiency increases dietary iron absorption, which is likely a compensatory mechanism to increase mitochondrial iron production.

Adults should follow the RDA of 900 mcg (1,000 mcg for pregnant women, 1,300 mcg for lactating women).

Iron

Iron is a large part of hemoglobin. Iron is also part of myoglobin, which helps muscle cells store oxygen. Without enough iron, ATP cannot be properly synthesized. As a result, some iron-deficient people become fatigued even when their hemoglobin levels are normal. Although iron is part of the antioxidant enzyme catalase, iron is not generally considered an antioxidant because too much iron can cause oxidative damage.

The most absorbable form of iron, called "heme" iron, is found in oysters, meat, poultry, and fish. Non-heme iron, which is absorbed less easily, is also found in these foods, as well as in dried fruit, molasses, leafy green vegetables, and wine. Acidic foods (such as tomato sauce) cooked in an iron pan can also become a source of dietary iron.

Normal aging of the brain and certain neurodegenerative changes share pathological and physiological changes with the retina, including mitochondrial dysfunction, oxidative stress, and loss of iron balance. It is becoming clear, in fact, that many organs show morphologic, physiologic, and biochemical changes before hemoglobin levels change. Heme is synthesized in the mitochondria and the decline in synthesis could explain the loss of iron in aging.

Vegetarians eat less iron than non-vegetarians and the iron they eat is less absorbable. As a result, vegetarians are more likely to have reduced iron stores. Iron deficiency, however, is not usually caused by a lack of iron in diet alone; an underlying cause, such as iron loss due to menstruation, often exists.

Several factors can lead to iron deficiency, including pregnancy, marathon running, parasitic infection, hemorrhoids, ulcers, ulcerative colitis, Crohn's disease, gastrointestinal cancer, and other conditions that cause blood loss or malabsorption. People who fit into one of these groups, however, shouldn't automatically take iron supplements. Fatigue, the first symptom of iron deficiency, may be caused by many other things. A nutritionist should assess the need for iron supplementation, since taking iron when it isn't required does no good and may do some harm.

If a lab test confirms iron deficiency, iron supplementation is essential and the practitioner must also determine the cause. Usually it's not serious (such as normal menstrual blood loss or blood donation).

Occasionally, however, iron deficiency signals ulcers or even colon cancer. Many premenopausal women become marginally iron deficient unless they supplement with iron. Even so, the 18 mg of iron present in most multivitamin supplements is often adequate.

An increase in consumption of iron can increase the risk of cardiac disease and retinal blood vessel issues. In general, most iron can be accumulated through a good diet, and the use of iron supplements is most often not needed.

The RDA of iron is 8 mg for adult males up to age fifty and 18 mg for adult females up to age fifty (27 mg for pregnant women, 9 mg for lactating women). For all adults fifty-one and over, the RDA is 8 mg.

Magnesium

Magnesium is an essential mineral that accounts for about .05 percent of the body's total weight. Nearly 70 percent of the body's supply is located in bone, together with calcium and phosphorus, while 30 percent is found in soft tissue and bodily fluids.

Magnesium is involved in many essential metabolic processes. Most of the body's magnesium is found inside the mitochondria, where it activates enzymes necessary for the metabolism of carbohydrates and amino acids. Moderate magnesium deficiency is common, particularly among African-Americans, and increases the risk of hypertension and diabetes. Evidence suggests that the balance between calcium and magnesium is especially important. If calcium consumption is high, magnesium intake must also be high. By countering the stimulating effect of calcium, magnesium plays an important role in neuromuscular contraction, mitigating conditions such as eyelid twitching.

The body's magnesium requirement is further influenced by the amounts of protein, phosphorus, and vitamin D in the diet. This requirement also increases when cholesterol levels are elevated or the consumption of protein is high. Magnesium helps to promote the absorption and metabolism of other minerals, as well as the utilization of B vitamins and vitamins C and E. It also helps to regulate the acid-alkaline balance in the body. It supports bone growth and is necessary for proper nerve and muscle function. Magnesium is also one of the minerals responsible for the conversion of essential fatty acids into DHA, the fatty acid most prominent in the brain and retina. It has also been shown to protect DNA, as the mineral is vital to telomerase activity. Telomerase is the enzyme responsible for telomere lengthening, a phenomenon associated with longevity and cell vitality.

Many foods contain magnesium, but it is found chiefly in fresh green vegetables, where it is an essential element of chlorophyll. Other excellent sources are raw wheat germ, soybeans, figs, corn, apples, and oil-rich seeds and nuts, especially almonds. It is estimated that the typical American diet provides about 120 mg of daily magnesium. Large amounts of magnesium can be toxic, especially if calcium intake is low and phosphorus intake is high. Excessive magnesium is usually excreted adequately, but in the event of kidney failure, there is a greater danger of toxicity because the rate of excretion is much lower.

Magnesium deficiency occurs most commonly in alcoholics, diabetics, sufferers of pancreatitis or kidney malfunction, and followers of high-carbohydrate diets. A deficiency is related to coronary heart disease, since it results in the formation of clots in the heart and brain, and may contribute to calcium deposits. Symptoms of deficiency include apprehensiveness, muscle twitching, tremors, confusion, and disorientation. Magnesium deficiency may also be a factor in endothelial dysfunction, which can lead to the development of atherosclerosis.

The RDA of magnesium for adult males up to the age of thirty is 400 mg, increasing to 420 mg for those over thirty. The RDA of magnesium for adult females up to the age of thirty is 310 mg (350 for pregnant women, 310 mg for lactating women), increasing to 320 mg for those thirty-one and over (360 mg for pregnant women, 320 mg for lactating women).

Manganese

Manganese is needed for healthy skin, bone, and cartilage formation, and plays a role in glucose tolerance. Inadequate manganese levels increase mitochondrial oxidants and subsequent mitochondrial decay.

Manganese deficiencies are rare. Individuals with osteoporosis sometimes have low blood levels of manganese suggestive of deficiency. Low levels of manganese can be associated with impaired glucose tolerance, as well as altered carbohydrate and fat metabolism.

Manganese is found in nuts, wheat germ, wheat bran, leafy green vegetables, beet greens, pineapple, and seeds.

Whether most people would benefit from manganese supplementation remains unclear. Amounts found in supplements (2 to 10 mg) have not been linked with toxicity, but excessive intake of manganese can lead to the rare side effects of dementia and psychiatric symptoms. Research suggests that individuals with cirrhosis may not be able to excrete manganese properly. Until more is known, these people should not supplement with manganese. Several minerals, such as calcium and iron, and possibly zinc, reduce the absorption of manganese. Zinc, copper, and manganese aid in the formation of superoxide dismutase—an important antioxidant enzyme.

The RDA of manganese is 2.3 mg for adult males and 1.8 mg for adult females (2.6 mg for pregnant women, 2 mg for lactating women).

Potassium

Potassium is one of the most common elements by mass in the human body. The body has about as much potassium as it has sulfur and chlorine, and only the major minerals calcium and phosphorus are more abundant.

Potassium plays an important part in the function of neurons and influences osmotic balance between cells and interstitial fluid. It also prevents muscle contraction. A shortage of potassium in the body may cause a potentially fatal condition known as hypokalemia, which typically results from vomiting, diarrhea, or increased urination. Deficiency symptoms include muscle weakness, paralytic ileus, ECG abnormalities, decreased reflex response, and, in severe cases, respiratory paralysis, alkalosis, and cardiac arrhythmia.

Clear cases of potassium deficiency are rare in healthy individuals. Foods rich in potassium include parsley, dried apricots, dried milk, chocolate, various nuts (especially almonds and pistachios), potatoes, bamboo shoots, bananas, avocados, soybeans, and bran, although it is also present in sufficient quantities in most fruits, vegetables, meat, and fish.

Studies in animals subject to hypertension indicate that diets high in potassium can reduce the risk of hypertension and possibly stroke (by a mechanism independent of blood pressure), while potassium deficiency combined with inadequate thiamine intake has produced heart disease in rats.

Individuals suffering from kidney disease may suffer adverse health effects from consuming large quantities of dietary potassium. Patients undergoing therapy by renal dialysis must observe strict dietary limits on potassium, as the kidneys control potassium excretion, and a buildup of potassium (hyperkalemia) may trigger fatal cardiac arrhythmia.

The recommended daily intake of potassium is 4.7 g for adults (5.1 g for pregnant women).

Selenium

Selenium is an essential mineral found in minute amounts in the body. It works closely with vitamin E in some of its metabolic actions, and in the promotion of normal body growth and fertility. Selenium is a natural antioxidant and, in particular, appears to preserve the elasticity of tissue as an antioxidant of polyunsaturated fatty acids, which can cause solidification of tissue proteins.

Selenium is found in the bran and germ of cereals, in vegetables such as broccoli, onions, and tomatoes, and in tuna. The amount of selenium in the liver and kidneys is approximately five times higher than that in muscle. Selenium is normally excreted in the urine. Its presence in the feces is an indication of improper absorption.

The recommended daily allowance of selenium for adults is extremely minute. This is due to the tendency of selenium to replace sulfur in biological compounds and inhibit the action of some enzymes. Selenium can be toxic in its pure form, so supplements should be taken with care. While low doses of selenium are considered useful in the prevention of cataract, higher doses have actually been found to induce them. An increased risk of cancer and a weakened immune system have also been associated with selenium deficiency.

As selenium preserves tissue elasticity, a lack of this mineral may encourage premature aging. This is of major significance for the crystalline lens, which becomes less flexible with age.

The RDA of selenium is 55 mcg for adults (60 mcg for pregnant women, 70 mcg for lactating women).

Sodium

Sodium is found predominantly in extracellular fluids, including vascular fluids within blood vessels and interstitial fluids surrounding cells. The remaining sodium in the body is found within the bones. Sodium works with potassium to equalize the acid-alkaline balance of the blood and regulate water levels within the body. Sodium and potassium are also involved in muscle contraction and expansion, as well as nerve stimulation. Another important function of sodium is keeping other minerals soluble so that they do not form deposits in the bloodstream. It helps to purge carbon dioxide from the body, supports digestion, and functions in the production of hydrochloric acid in the stomach. In addition, it acts with chlorine to improve blood and lymph health.

Sodium is found in virtually all foods, and obviously in table salt as sodium chloride. High concentrations are found in seafood, carrots, beets, poultry, and meat. Kelp can be an excellent supplemental source of sodium in the diet.

There is no established dietary requirement for sodium, but it is generally understood that the usual intake far exceeds need. The average American has a total sodium intake of between 9 and 25 g per day. An excess of sodium in the diet may cause potassium to be lost in the urine. Abnormal fluid retention accompanied by dizziness and swelling of the legs or face may also occur. Diets containing excessive amounts of sodium also contribute to an increase in blood pressure. The simplest way to reduce sodium intake is to eliminate table salt and reduce bread consumption in the diet.

The Food and Drug Administration recommends a daily intake of no more than 2.3 g. People over fifty, as well as those with ailments such as diabetes or kidney disease, should ingest no more than 1.5 g per day.

Zinc

Zinc is an essential trace mineral that occurs in the body in a larger amount than any other trace element except iron. The human body contains approximately 1.8 g of zinc, compared to nearly 5 g of iron.

Zinc has a variety of functions. It is related to the normal absorption and action of vitamins, especially vitamin A and the B complex. It is a constituent of at least twenty-five enzymes involved in digestion and metabolism. It is a component of insulin and the enzyme needed to break down alcohol. It also plays a role in carbohydrate digestion and phosphorus metabolism. It has an important function in general growth and development, the operation of the prostate gland, the healing of wounds and burns, and the synthesis of DNA.

Zinc, like magnesium, is a powerful anti-inflammatory mineral, although it is known primarily for its role in improving the function and performance of the immune system. Zinc becomes more important as people age, since immune dysfunction and inflammation become more pronounced and problematic over the years.

The best source of all trace elements in proper balance is natural, unprocessed food, especially food grown in organically enriched soil. Diets high in protein, whole grain products, brewer's yeast, wheat bran, wheat germ, and pumpkin seeds are usually high in zinc.

Zinc is relatively nontoxic, although poisoning may result from eating food that has been stored in a galvanized container. High intakes of zinc interfere with copper utilization, causing incomplete iron metabolism. It is important to note that when zinc is added to the diet, vitamin A is also needed in larger amounts.

Many supplements use zinc oxide in their formulas. This is the least biologically active and most difficult to absorb form of zinc, and it must be combined with the proper amount of copper to avoid severe reaction. Monomethionine zinc is the most bioavailable form of zinc, and the only form that does not interfere with copper absorption.

The RDA of zinc is 11 mg for adult males and 8 mg for adult females (11 mg for pregnant women, 12 mg for lactating women). The consensus recommendation is 25mg, with a maximum of 40 mg.

OTHER HELPFUL SUBSTANCES

As you now know, many macronutrients and micronutrients are crucial to good health and, more specifically, to good eye health. In addition to the vitamins, minerals, and other compounds recently discussed, there are a number of natural substances that should be considered for optimal well-being and vision care.

Acetyl-L-Carnitine (ALC)

Acetyl-L-carnitine is a form of the amino acid L-carnitine. It delivers omega-3 long-chain fatty acids to the mitochondria and transports small-chain and medium-chain fatty acids out of the mitochondria in order to maintain normal coenzyme A levels within cells. This is particularly important in the maintenance of retina health, due to the large number of mitochondria within retinal cells.

ALC levels may decrease with advancing age, but because it is not an essential nutrient, true deficiency does not occur. Most research involving acetyl-L-carnitine has used supplements of 500 mg three times a day, while some research has used double this amount. Side effects from taking acetyl-L-carnitine are uncommon, though skin rash, increased appetite, nausea, vomiting, agitation, and body odor have been reported in people taking excessive amounts.

An ALC intake of 200 mg daily is recommended.

Bioflavonoids

Bioflavonoids, once known as vitamin P, are water-soluble and composed of a group of brightly colored substances that often appear in fruits and vegetables with vitamin C. Bioflavonoids were first discovered in the white part between the rind and the fruit of citrus species. In fact, the edible part of citrus fruit contains ten times more bioflavonoids than the juice. Sources of bioflavonoids include lemons, grapes, plums, black currants, grapefruits, apricots, buckwheat, cherries, blackberries, and rose hips.

Bioflavonoids help the body to absorb and use vitamin C. They assist vitamin C in keeping collagen healthy. They also have the ability to increase the strength of capillaries and regulate their permeability. These actions help to prevent hemorrhages and ruptures in capillaries and connective tissue, and to build a protective barrier against infection. Retinal hemorrhages may be reduced to some degree through the use of vitamin C-bioflavonoid supplementation. While bioflavonoids have not proven to have the antioxidant abilities once attributed to them, they seem to chelate (bind) iron and copper ions to specific proteins, which limits the production of free radicals. This could be very beneficial to AMD patients. In addition, many of the biological effects of bioflavonoids are related to their ability to modulate cell-signaling pathways. This activity is very important to those at higher risk of genetic degenerative disease, including AMD and Alzheimer's.

The absorption and storage properties, daily requirements, deficiency symptoms, and bodily utilization of bioflavonoids are all similar to those of vitamin C.

Carotenoids

Carotenoids are fat-soluble yellow, orange, or red pigments found predominantly in plants. While there are several subclassifications of carotenoids, the most familiar to eyecare professionals are provitamin A carotenoids and non-provitamin A carotenoids—in other words, those that can and those that cannot be converted into vitamin A. To date, over 600 carotenoids have been identified in nature, and these are produced by plants, algae, and bacteria. Animals appear to be incapable of biosynthesizing carotenoids but use them for a variety of purposes, including coloration, and so must obtain them from food. Only two commonly ingested carotenoids have been found in the retina: lutein and zeaxanthin. A third carotenoid, mesozeaxanthin, is also found in the central retina but not routinely taken in through the diet.

Carotenoids lutein, zeaxanthin, and mesozeaxanthin are macular pigments, which appear as a yellow tint. The intense deposition of these yellow pigments in and around the part of the eye called the *fovea centralis* provides the basis for the clinical description of this area as the *macula lutea,* or yellow spot. These carotenoids perform two primary functions in connection with this area. First, they filter high-energy blue wavelengths of visible light before they reach the photoreceptors. By passively absorbing these wavelengths, these macular pigments limit photo-oxidative damage to tissue. Second, these macular pigments function as antioxidants to directly protect the retina from damage caused by reactive oxygen species. In other words, macular pigment may be characterized as "internal sunglasses" for the eyes.

The ability of macular pigment to absorb or filter blue light is measured as macular pigment optical density (MPOD). MPOD is an optical indicator of the concentration of lutein and zeaxanthin in the macula and is becoming an accepted way of determining not only the risk of eye disease but also visual function. The degree of increase in MPOD following lutein or zeaxanthin supplementation varies, likely due to differences in subject demographics, disease states, diets, supplementation regimens, or other factors. Supplementation of up to 140 mg per day has been studied and has not shown any negative effects.

Macular pigment, likely via its ability to filter blue light, has been shown to enhance visual performance. High levels of macular pigment contribute to improvements in visual acuity, glare tolerance and recovery, contrast sensitivity, and photophobia in healthy individuals as well as those diagnosed with age-related eye disease. There is a growing body of evidence that suggests low levels of MPOD may be a risk factor in certain age-related eye conditions. Increased MPOD may provide greater protection against oxidative damage, which contributes to the manifestation of AMD. For example, risk factors for AMD, including tobacco use, light iris color, advanced age, obesity, and being female are also associated with low levels of MPOD.

In addition to being present in the macula, lutein and zeaxanthin are also deposited in the lens, albeit at much lower concentrations. The fact that oxidation of the lens is the major cause of cataract suggests that antioxidant nutrients may play a role in cataract prevention. Findings show that lutein may also affect immune response and inflammation. Since AMD has features of a chronic low-grade systemic inflammatory response, attention to the exact role of lutein in this disease has shifted from a local effect in the eye towards a possible systemic anti-inflammatory function.

Lutein and zeaxanthin are found naturally together in vegetables such as spinach, kale, broccoli, corn, green peas, and green beans, as well as other foods, including egg yolks. The bioavailability of lutein is actually enhanced by chopping and cooking the source food. It is difficult, however, to obtain beneficial amounts of lutein and zeaxanthin through diet alone. Lutein and zeaxanthin are related due to their very similar chemical structures. Zeaxanthin is one of the most common carotenoid alcohols found in nature. It is the pigment that gives paprika (made from bell peppers) and saffron their unmistakeably red color. Spirulina is also a rich source of zeaxanthin and can serve as a dietary supplement. Several observational studies have connected high dietary intake of foods containing zeaxanthin with lower incidence of AMD.

Mesozeaxanthin is found in the retina, but unlike lutein and zeaxanthin, it has not been isolated from the liver and is not produced within the body or derived from the traditional American diet. Mesozeaxanthin is primarily absorbed through natural conversion of enzymes from lutein. It is a powerful antioxidant, allowing even greater blue-light filtration than the previously mentioned carotenoids. Some research suggests that, for a small percentage of the population, natural enzyme conversion of lutein into mesozeaxanthin may not be sufficient. For these patients, supplementation of mesozeaxanthin directly fortifies pigment density in the central macula without known adverse side effects. Due to this substance's biochemical properties, all supplements of mesozeaxanthin are combined with lutein and zeaxanthin.

Interventional studies report that 10 mg of lutein per day is effective in improving vision and reducing the risk of certain eye conditions. A survey of the standard American diet showed an approximate daily intake of 2 mg of lutein. Most authorities recommend 15 to 20 mg of lutein daily. Although there is no recommended dietary allowance of zeaxanthin, approximately 8 mg daily is the suggested amount for anyone diagnosed with macular degeneration, while 2 to 4 mg is an appropriate amount for those taking it as a preventative measure.

Lycopene is another important pigment. It is responsible for the bright colors of certain fruits and vegetables, performs various functions in photosynthesis, and protects certain organisms from excessive light damage. Lycopene is a key intermediate in the biosynthesis of many important carotenoids, including beta-carotene and xanthophylls. Given this connection to beta-carotene and xanthophylls, many sources suggest it is critical to eye health. There is no lycopene found in the eye, however, and any positive effect of this carotenoid to ocular health is secondary.

Astaxanthin is a unique carotenoid that is ubiquitous in marine ecosystems. Originating in aquatic microorganisms and microalgae, astaxanthin lends red and pink coloration to higher organisms such as krill, shrimp, and salmon. Among carotenoids, astaxanthin is distinguished by a unique chemical structure, two extra hydroxyl groups. This attribute affords a tenfold greater antioxidant capacity than other carotenoids, including beta-carotene and lutein. In addition to being an antioxidant powerhouse, astaxanthin modulates nuclear factor kappa B (NFkB), which controls the inflammatory response of almost every cell, including those comprising the immune system, connective tissue, vascular system, adipose tissue, eyes, and skin.

Coenzyme Q_{10} (COQ_{10})

Coenzyme Q_{10}, or CoQ_{10}, is a fat-soluble compound primarily synthesized by the body but also consumed through diet. It is required for mitochondrial energy synthesis, thus a high concentration is found in the inner membrane of the mitochondria. The primary role of CoQ_{10} is as a catalyst for metabolism. It also functions as an antioxidant in cell membranes and lipoproteins. Acting in conjunction with enzymes, CoQ_{10} speeds up the metabolic process, providing the energy cells need to digest food, heal wounds, maintain healthy muscles, and perform countless other bodily functions. It is especially abundant in the energy-intensive cells of the heart and retina.

CoQ_{10} acts as an antioxidant, much like vitamins C and E, helping to neutralize cell-damaging free radicals. It may play a role in preventing cancer, heart attack, and other diseases linked to free-radical damage. It's also used as a general energy enhancer and anti-aging supplement. Supplementation helps to boost energy and overall cognitive function. Because levels of this compound diminish with age (and with certain diseases), some doctors recommend daily supplementation beginning at age forty.

The synthesis of an intermediary precursor of coenzyme Q_{10}, mevalonate, is inhibited by some beta blockers, blood pressure-lowering medication, and statins. Statins can reduce serum levels of CoQ_{10} by up to 40 percent, in fact. Therefore, CoQ_{10} supplements should be routinely

Free Radicals and Antioxidants

All antioxidants operate in a similar manner in the body and play an important role in its basic defense system against disease, infection, premature aging, and possibly the adverse effects of strenuous athletic performance.

At the root of many diseases and the aging process are a group of highly reactive substances known as free radicals or oxidants, which are also classified as reactive oxygen species, or ROS. These chemical compounds consist of two or more elements along with an unpaired, or extra, electron. This unpaired electron makes the compound reactive and unstable—a free radical. To stabilize itself, the free radical seeks out and grabs an electron from a stable compound, creating a new free radical and staring a chain reaction. In this way, free radicals attack cell components and cause damage to cells and tissues in the body. Common sites of attack are polyunsaturated fatty acids in cell membranes. Free-radical-induced damage alters cell-membrane structure and function. The membrane is no longer able to transport nutrients, oxygen, or water into the cell, or to regulate the removal of waste products. Continued free-radical attack ruptures the cell membrane, causing a loss of cellular components and rendering the cell useless. Free radicals also damage the mitochondria, which results in limit-

taken if statin drugs are being used—typically 100 mg of CoQ_{10} per 20-mg dose of statins. For general recommended daily intake, 30 mg of CoQ_{10} should be adequate.

Hyaluronic Acid

Hyaluronic acid, or hyaluronan, is found in numerous parts of the body, including skin, cartilage, and the vitreous humor. Therefore, it is well suited to biomedical applications targeting these areas. The first hyaluronan biomedical product, known by the brand name Healon (sodium hyaluronate), was initially developed in the 1970s by Pharmacia, and is now used in numerous types of eye surgery (corneal transplantation, cataract surgery, glaucoma surgery, and retinal detachment repair). Other biomedical companies also produce brands of hyaluronan for ophthalmic surgery. Since its initial biomedical usage, hyaluronic acid has benefited an estimated quarter of a billion patients during eye surgery thanks to its useful properties.

ed or halted production of energy for all processes of the cell. Free-radical damage to enzymes and other proteins limits the building of tissue and causes accumulation of protein fragments. Finally, a cell cannot reproduce normally when its genetic code has been altered by free radicals. At best, the cell dies. At worst, the cell mutates into a cancerous cell. This destructive process is, in fact, associated with the initiation of numerous disorders, from arthritis to cardiovascular disease.

Free radicals, however, are unavoidable. They are formed during normal metabolic processes. They also are obtained from some foods, inhaled with polluted air and tobacco smoke, and generated in the environment by radiation and herbicides. Fortunately, the body can defend against free-radicals with antioxidants, including enzymes such as superoxide dismutase (SOD) and glutathione peroxidase; vitamins such as C and E; carotenoids such as beta-carotene; minerals such as zinc and selenium; herbs such as bilberry and ginkgo; and other nutrients such as cysteine, pine bark extract, coenzyme Q_{10}, and bioflavonoids. These substances intercede, deactivating free radicals and rendering them harmless before they can cause irreversible damage. They are currently being investigated for their role in the prevention of many major diseases, including eye conditions such as cataract and AMD.

Since hyaluronan holds water so well, it has been suggested to be used to supplement the vitreous humor in cases of vitreous detachment. The human eye loses hyaluronic acid as it ages, so supplementation is likely a good course. Other nutritional factors such as echinacea, grapeseed extract, inositol hexaphosphate, and quercetin can help to stabilize hyaluronan and possibly prevent its breakdown.

At this time, there is no recommended amount of hyaluronic acid for daily intake. In adults over the age of eighteen, 50 mg of hyaluronic acid have been taken by mouth once or twice daily with meals as supplementation. Dry eye has been treated with 0.2-percent hyaluronic acid eye drops three to four times daily for three months.

Lactoferrin

Lactoferrin (LF) is an iron-binding protein found in milk. It is the main glycoprotein component of the watery layer of the tear film. Lactoferrin has many functions in the eye, including having anti-inflammatory effects, balancing tear-film lipocalin, and inhibiting bacterial biofilm formation on the ocular surface. Lactoferrin, structurally similar to transferrin, is also known as lactotransferrin (LTF), a protein with antimicrobial activity that is part of the body's innate defense system. Transferrin is found in the mucosa and binds iron, creating an environment low in free iron. This impedes bacterial survival in a process called iron withholding.

Oral lactoferrin avoids absorption in the stomach through digestive conversion into a very small molecule called lactoferricin, which is then transported into secretory tissues, including the lacrimal gland, which is responsible for secreting the watery layer the tear film. Lactoferrin is also produced in the lacrimal gland by white blood cells as the first line of defense against infection.

In one study, oral lactoferrin supplementation reduced inflammatory levels and other biochemical factors associated with induced dry eye syndrome in mice. In a recent Chinese study, acupuncture increased lactoferrin levels in tears of patients with dry eye. In another study, fasting was shown to decrease tear proteins and enzymes, suggesting that nutritional deficiencies affect the entire body, including tear film biochemistry and visual acuity.

Unfortunately, most oral products designed to address the lipid layer of the tear film do not address tear film stability, biochemical balance, or nutritional function of natural tears.

Treatment of dry eye can be effective with 10 mg of lactoferrin per day.

Lipoic Acid

Lipoic acid is both water-soluble and fat-soluble, and is a vital cofactor in the production of enzymes necessary for proper mitochondrial function. Alpha-lipoic acid (ALA), not to be confused with the fatty acid alpha-linoleic acid (ALA), works together with other antioxidants, such as vitamins C and E. It is important for growth, aids in the prevention of cell damage, and helps the body to rid itself of harmful toxins.

Several studies suggest that treatment with ALA may reduce pain, burning, itching, tingling, and numbness in people who have peripheral neuropathy caused by diabetes. Alpha-lipoic acid has been used for years for this purpose in Europe. Other studies have shown that ALA speeds the removal of glucose from the blood of people with diabetes, and that this antioxidant may prevent kidney damage associated with diabetes in animals.

ALA may prove useful in the treatment of chronic hepatitis because it relieves stress on the liver and helps to rid the body of toxins. There have been several case reports of the use of ALA in combination with silymarin (milk thistle) and selenium (a substance with liver-protective and anti-oxidant properties) to treat hepatitis C.

Because ALA can pass easily into the brain, it has protective effects on brain and nerve tissues, and shows promise as a treatment for stroke and other brain disorders involving free-radical damage. In one study, animals treated with ALA suffered less brain damage and had greater survival rates after stroke than animals that had not received this supplement. While animal studies are encouraging, more research is needed to understand whether this benefit applies to people as well. And, of course, anything that's good for the brain is good for the retina.

ALA may also prove useful in conditions such as heart failure, HIV, cataract, and glaucoma. More research is underway in these areas. Good food sources of alpha-lipoic acid include spinach, broccoli, beef, brewer's yeast, and certain organ meats (such as kidneys and heart).

While there is no established RDA for ALA, 150 mg seems to be an adequate daily intake.

Pycnogenol

Pycnogenol is a French maritime pine bark extract. The ingredient is available in more than 700 dietary supplements, multivitamins, and food and beverage products worldwide. Besides possessing potent and unique antioxidant properties, pycnogenol is a water-soluble compound representing a natural combination of procyanidins, bioflavonoids, and organic acids. Pycnogenol has four basic properties: It is a powerful antioxidant, acts as a natural anti-inflammatory, selectively binds to collagen and elastin, and aids in the production of endothelial nitric oxide, which helps to dilate blood vessels.

Close to 300 scientific articles and clinical trials have confirmed pycnogenol's safety, absence of toxicity, and clinical efficacy over the past forty years. Published findings have demonstrated pycnogenol's beneficial health effects in cardiovascular and circulatory health, joint health, skin care, blood glucose balance, eye health (specifically glaucoma), and sports nutrition.

Resveratrol

No discussion of eye health would be complete without mentioning the supposed "super-molecule" of nutrition: Resveratrol. Resveratrol was originally isolated from the roots of hellebore plants in 1940 by Takaoka, and later, in 1963, from the roots of Japanese knotweed. It attracted wider attention only in 1992, however, when its presence in wine was suggested as the explanation for the cardioprotective effects of this beverage.

The resveratrol in grapes is contained mainly in the skin and protects against the growth of fungal pathogens. The resveratrol content of wine is highly influenced, in fact, by the amount of time it spends in contact with the skins of the grapes used in production. Red wine actually has very little reseveratrol.

The effects of resveratrol are currently the topic of numerous animal and human studies. Its impact on lifespan remains controversial, with uncertain effects in fruit flies, nematode worms, and short-lived fish. Anticancer, anti-inflammatory, blood sugar-lowering, and beneficial cardiovascular effects have been reported in mouse and rat experiments. In humans, however, resveratrol may have fewer benefits. In one positive human trial, extremely high doses (3 to 5 g) of resveratrol (in a proprietary formulation designed to enhance its bioavailability) significantly lowered blood sugar, but this study has never been published in a peer-reviewed scientific publication. Studies have shown that resveratrol possesses blood sugar-lowering effects on diabetic rats, improving common symptoms of this condition. Other diabetic animal model studies by a number of different researchers have also demonstrated these fascinating antidiabetic effects of resveratrol.

Despite the mainstream press alleging resveratrol's anti-aging effects, there are no accepted data to form a scientific basis for the application of these claims to mammals. At the present time, research on resveratrol is in its infancy and the long-term effects of supplementation in humans are not known. Resveratrol is likely safe when used in the amounts found in some foods, but during pregnancy and breastfeeding, the source of resveratrol is important. Resveratrol is found in grape skins, grape juice, wine, and other food sources, but, of course, wine should not be used as a source of resveratrol during pregnancy or breastfeeding.

In connection with hormone-sensitive conditions such as breast cancer, uterine cancer, ovarian cancer, endometriosis, and uterine fibroids, resveratrol might act as an estrogen. If you have any condition that might be made worse by exposure to estrogen, don't supplement with resveratrol. It may also increase the risk of bleeding during and after surgery. In light of this information, patients should stop using resveratrol at least two weeks before a scheduled surgery.

In direct use for eye conditions, a clinical study at the Veterans Health Center in North Chicago, Illinois, was conducted to see if a commercial resveratrol product, Longevinex, could rescue the sight of patients who had failed medical therapy and had no other options available. Researchers reported that sixteen of the first seventeen patients treated with the product displayed measurable visual improvement, some experiencing rapid and dramatic restoration of functional vision (vision good enough to drive a car or thread a needle).

EYE STRUCTURES AND SUPPORTIVE NUTRIENTS

While there is no simple method to account for which nutrients support which parts of the eye, some nutrients are known to be more prominent than others in certain areas of the eye. The following is a general list of this information.

EYE STRUCTURES AND SUPPORTIVE NUTRIENTS	
Eye Structure	Nutrient
Aqueous humor	Glutathione, lutein, vitamin C, vitamin E, zeaxanthin.
Cornea	CoQ_{10}, collagen, hyaluronic acid.
Crystalline lens	Glutathione, lutein, potassium, vitamin C, vitamin E, zeaxanthin.
Optic nerve	Glutathione, vitamin B_2, vitamin B_{12}.
Photoreceptors	DHA, vitamin A, zinc.
Retinal pigmented epithelium	Selenium, vitamin E.
Retinal nerve layer	Glutathione, hyaluronic acid, lutein, zeaxanthin.
Sclera	Collagen, hyaluronic acid, iron, proline, vitamin C.
Tear film	Essential fatty acids, lactoferrin, vitamin A.
Vitreous humor	Antioxidants, hyaluronic acid, selenium, vitamin C, water.

Always remember, however, that nutrients work together to support the visual system.

USING CAUTION

Most herbs and supplements have not been thoroughly tested for interactions with other herbs, supplements, drugs, or foods. Always read product labels before trying any supplement of any kind. In addition, if you have a medical condition or are taking other drugs, herbs, or supplements, you should consult with your primary healthcare provider before starting any new therapy.

PART TWO

Eye Problems

While not every eye condition may be improved through nutritional intervention, most diseases and disorders need a healthy body to combat illness appropriately. People with well-supported immune systems heal faster and better. It is that simple. When it comes to your vision, it is important to know common eye concerns and learn which nutritional supplements, herbal therapies, or homeopathic remedies may be used to treat them.

ACCOMMODATIVE INSUFFICIENCY

The ability to focus on objects at various distances requires the power of the eye to vary. This modification of focusing power is called accommodation. Accommodation strength gradually decreases with age, but this decrease is typically not noticed until the age of about forty years old. Any loss of accommodative ability before the age of forty is considered abnormal and called accommodative insufficiency. This condition is most commonly seen in school-aged children who have difficulty focusing on their reading materials.

This issue is typically thought of as a loss of strength of the eye muscles and their ability to focus the eyes properly. There are two kinds of muscles in the body: the "smooth" type, which are under automatic control, and the "striated" type, which are under intentional control. Both types play roles in eye movement and are controlled by nerves, so nutrients that support nerves and muscles are important to maintaining adequate accommodation.

While nutrients to address accommodative insufficiency are not normally recommended, they can support smooth and striated muscles, as well as increase oxygen utilization.

NUTRITIONAL SUPPLEMENTS

Supplement	Directions for Use	Comments
Astaxanthin	6 mg daily.	Protects cell membrane components from oxidative stress and inflammation.
Calcium	600 mg daily.	Should be balanced with equal amounts of phosphorus and magnesium.
Vitamin B_2 (riboflavin)	75 mg daily.	Good for nerves, muscles, and eye fatigue.
Vitamin C	250 mg 4 times daily.	Nourishes the lens.
Vitamin E	200 IU daily.	Antioxidant.

HOMEOPATHIC REMEDIES

Remedy	Directions for Use	Comments
Cocculus 6c	3 to 4 pellets under the tongue 3 to 4 times daily.	Good for accommodative insufficiency associated with nausea.

Remedy	Directions for Use	Comments
Gelsemium sempervirens 6c	3 to 4 pellets under the tongue 3 to 4 times daily.	Good for accommodative insufficiency associated with headache.
Natrum muriaticum 6c	3 to 4 pellets under the tongue 3 to 4 times daily.	Good for accommodative insufficiency associated with anger or irritability.

ARCUS SENILIS

Arcus senilis refers to an opaque white, blue, or grey ring that forms around the periphery of the cornea. It most often develops during later years, but is not uncommon in middle age or even younger. It has been known to occur in black patients about a decade earlier than in white patients. It is more common in men and may be associated with dyslipidemia, decreased omega-3 intake, alcohol, high blood pressure, diabetes, smoking, xanthalasma, and coronary heart disease.

Arcus senilis may be a valuable indication of the state of fat and cholesterol metabolism. According to Dr. Stuart Richer, this condition is a known biometric indicator of biologic aging and mortality, especially in males, offering insight into the health of the cardiovascular system. It is also associated with vitamin D and magnesium deficiencies. The general consensus is that arcus senilis is normal in older adults, but can be a sign of elevated cholesterol in middle-aged or younger individuals, particularly those with the genetic variant of familial hyperlipidemia. Efforts should be made to reduce triglycerides through the use of omega-3 fatty acids, and to normalize vitamin D and magnesium levels.

NUTRITIONAL SUPPLEMENTS

Supplement	Directions for Use	Comments
Chromium picolinate	400 to 600 mcg daily.	Lowers cholesterol levels and improves HDL-LDL ratio.
L-carnitine	1,000 mg 3 times daily with meals.	Supports cholesterol metabolism, liver function and gallbladder function, and transports essential fatty acids.
Lecithin	1,200 mg 3 times daily before meals.	Emulsifies fat in the body.

Supplement	Directions for Use	Comments
Niacin	Up to 1,000 mg extended-release form daily. (Taking it before bedtime with food will reduce flushing.)	Raises HDL cholesterol.
Phosphatide	1,500 mg daily.	Emulsifies fat in the body.
Vitamin D$_3$	2,000 to 4,000 IU daily.	Supports the immune system.

HERBS AND HERBAL SUPPLEMENTS

Herb	Directions for Use	Comments
Garlic	As directed on label.	Reduces cholesterol levels.
Ginger	As directed on label.	Reduces cholesterol levels.

BLEPHARITIS

Blepharitis is inflammation of the eyelids that usually causes symptoms of itching, irritation, burning, and a foreign body sensation in the eye. It sometimes includes red eyelids with ulcerations that may bleed. Vision is usually normal, although a poor tear film often causes intermittent blurriness.

Prevention and treatment of this condition go hand in hand. For people who suffer from the condition, regular eye hygiene is the best way to prevent outbreaks. In addition, warm compresses should be applied three to four times a day. One of the most common of these techniques is to use a teabag as a warm compress, but a washcloth soaked in warm water works just as well. The natural astringent factor of tea will help to soften oils that may be trapped in ducts. The eyelids should also be massaged in a circular motion to loosen debris.

Nutrients that support healthy skin are helpful in the treatment of blepharitis, as are nutrients that support healthy oil production.

NUTRITIONAL SUPPLEMENTS

Supplement	Directions for Use	Comments
Vitamin A	3,000 IU daily.	Good for dry skin.
Vitamin B complex	75 mg daily.	Promotes healthy skin and proper circulation. Aids in cellular reproduction.

Supplement	Directions for Use	Comments
Vitamin C with bioflavonoids	6,000 mg daily in divided doses. (Use powdered buffered ascorbic acid.)	Antioxidant that reduces inflammation.
Zinc (monomethionine)	25 mg daily. (Do not take more than 40 mg daily.)	Enhances immune function.
Copper	1 mg daily with zinc.	Needed to balance zinc (if not monomethionine form).
Linoleic acid	500 mg daily. (Use black current seed oil.)	Supports skin tissue.
Omega-3 fish oil	2,000 mg daily.	Supports gland secretions.

HERBS AND HERBAL SUPPLEMENTS

Herb	Directions for Use	Comments
Dulse	Apply as a compress.	High in iodine.
Goldenseal	Apply as a compress.	Soothes tissues. Do not use during pregnancy.
Horsetail	Apply as a compress.	Tones the skin.
Rosemary	Apply as a compress.	Stimulates the skin.
Sage	Apply as a compress.	Astringent.

HOMEOPATHIC REMEDIES

Remedy	Directions for Use	Comments
Antimonium crudum 6c	3 to 4 pellets under the tongue 3 to 4 times daily.	Good for all skin conditions.
Argentum nitricum 6c	3 to 4 pellets under the tongue 3 to 4 times daily.	Good for all skin conditions.
Arsenicum album 6c	3 to 4 pellets under the tongue 3 to 4 times daily.	Good for blepharitis associated with anxiety or burning.
Calcarea sulfurica 6c	3 to 4 pellets under the tongue 3 to 4 times daily.	Good for all skin conditions.
Carboneum sulfuratum 6c	3 to 4 pellets under the tongue 3 to 4 times daily.	Good for all skin conditions.

Remedy	Directions for Use	Comments
Euphrasia officinalis 6c	3 to 4 pellets under the tongue 3 to 4 times daily.	Good for blepharitis associated with soreness.
Graphites 6c	3 to 4 pellets under the tongue 3 to 4 times daily.	Good for all skin conditions.
Hepar sulphuris 6c	3 to 4 pellets under the tongue 3 to 4 times daily.	Good for all skin conditions.
Lycopodium 6c	3 to 4 pellets under the tongue 3 to 4 times daily.	Good for all skin conditions.
Petroleum 6c	3 to 4 pellets under the tongue 3 to 4 times daily.	Good for all skin conditions.
Rhus toxicodendron 6c	3 to 4 pellets under the tongue 3 to 4 times daily.	Good for all skin conditions.
Sulphur 6c	3 to 4 pellets under the tongue 3 to 4 times daily.	Good for all skin conditions.

RECOMMENDATIONS

- Do not rub your eyes, even if they feel itchy.

- Apply a warm compress to your eyes a few times a day for at least ten minutes each time. To enhance the effect, make a tea of your chosen herb, soak a clean cloth in the tea, and apply the cloth as your compress. When finished, gently wipe your eyelids with the compress to remove any excess debris. Never reuse a compress.

- Stay away from irritants, such as smoke, wind, excessive sunlight, and bright lights.

- Eat a well-balanced diet that emphasizes fresh raw vegetables, whole grains, legumes, and fresh fruits. Eliminate sugar.

- Get sufficient sleep and avoid eyestrain.

BLEPHAROSPASM

Blepharospasm is a dystonia—a disorder caused by abnormal involuntary sustained muscle contractions and spasms. Patients with blepharospasm have normal eyes; the visual disturbance is solely the repeated forced closure of the eyelids.

Blepharospasm's first sign is generally excessive blinking or eye irritation, sometimes happening during specific conditions such as bright lights, fatigue, or emotional tension. The spasms tend to disappear during sleep and may reappear only after a few hours of being awake. Concentrating on a task may diminish the problem, but over time, spasms may become blinding to the sufferer, whose eyelids may remain forcefully closed for several hours.

Conventional treatment consists of Botox, which is injected in minute doses into muscles above and below the eyes. Injections are usually given in the eyelid, brow, and muscles under the lower lid. The benefits begin one to fourteen days after treatment and last for an average of three to four months. Long-term follow-up studies have shown this treatment to be very safe and effective, with up to 90 percent of patients obtaining almost complete relief from their symptoms.

Magnesium helps muscles to function properly and relax. It keeps heart rhythm steady and supports a healthy immune system. Stress reduction is also recommended for patients with blepharospam. Meditation, breathing techniques, biofeedback, yoga, visualization, and counseling are all appropriate ways to lower stress. Acupuncture is also a viable alternative to traditional medical treatments for blepharospam.

NUTRITIONAL SUPPLEMENTS		
Supplement	Directions for Use	Comments
Calcium	1,000 mg daily.	For proper muscle function.
Folic acid	400 mcg daily.	For proper nerve production.
Magnesium	350 mg daily.	For muscle relaxation.
Phosphorus	800 mg daily.	For proper nerve growth.
Potassium	2,500 mg daily.	Rebalances the nerves.
Vitamin B complex	100 mg daily.	For stress.
Vitamin C with bioflavonoids	500 mg every 3 hours up to 4 times daily. (Use powdered buffered ascorbic acid.	Antioxidant.

HERBS AND HERBAL SUPPLEMENTS

Herb	Directions for Use	Comments
Lobelia	Apply as a compress.	Relieves muscle cramping. Do not take internally.
Valerian	2 to 4 grams daily.	For relaxation.

HOMEOPATHIC REMEDIES

Remedy	Directions for Use	Comments
Agaricus 6c	3 to 4 pellets under the tongue 3 to 4 times daily.	For eyelid twitching.
Calcarea carbonica 6c and Magnesia phosphorica 6c	3 to 4 pellets of each under the tongue 3 to 4 times daily.	For blepharospasm associated with mineral deficiency.
Hypericum perforatum 6c	3 to 4 pellets under the tongue 3 to 4 times daily.	For eyelid twitching.
Ignatia amara 6c	3 to 4 pellets under the tongue 3 to 4 times daily.	For eyelid twitching.
Nux vomica 6c	3 to 4 pellets under the tongue 3 to 4 times daily.	For eyelid spasm after drinking coffee.
Physostigma 6c	3 to 4 pellets under the tongue 3 to 4 times daily.	For eyelid twitching.
Rheum 6c	3 to 4 pellets under the tongue 3 to 4 times daily.	For eyelid twitching.
Sulphur 6c	3 to 4 pellets under the tongue 3 to 4 times daily.	For eyelid twitching.

CATARACT

Any loss of transparency in the crystalline lens of the eye is called a cataract. Cataracts are not limited to the aged, although cataracts more commonly appear in the older population. Between the ages of sixty-five and seventy-four, about 23 percent of the population is expected to have a cataract. After the age of seventy-five years old, about 50 percent of people will develop a cataract.

Epidemiologic studies suggest that cataract risk factors include age, sex, race, occupation, educational status, light iris color, diabetes mellitus, hypertension, drug exposure, smoking, and sunlight exposure. Deficiencies in vitamins C and E, carotenoids, and trace elements zinc and selenium may also be associated with the development of cataract. The lens can accumulate minerals such as iron, cadmium, calcium, and magnesium. This accumulation eventually leads to cataract formation. Smoking, in fact, increases iron levels in the lens.

Lutein and zeaxanthin might impact cataract risk. They are the only carotenoids in the human lens. Clinical findings show that lens optical density is inversely related to MPOD among adults between the ages of forty-eight and seventy-two years old. In addition, estrogen supplementation may reduce the risk of cataract formation. This process might be related to the modulation of HDL levels by estrogen in the blood.

Oxidative stress is as a major factor in cataract development. There have been many studies conducted on nutrition and cataract formation. It has been shown, for example, that diets low in vitamin B_2 can lead to cataract development. In horses, cataracts, which are a common cause of blindness in these animals, can be reduced when large amounts of vitamin B_2 are added to the diet. Coincidentally, galactose, a type of milk sugar, increases the need for vitamin B_2. In infants who cannot utilize galactose normally, poor vision from cataracts has been corrected by removing milk sugar from the diet and adding vitamin B_2.

A 1997 study found a significant reduction in cataract development in a group of nurses who took vitamin C supplements. In this study of 478 nurses, ages fifty-three to seventy-three years old, over a period of thirteen to fifteen years, high vitamin C intake protected against a certain form of cataract. Women using vitamin C supplements for ten years or more experienced a reduction in risk of 64 percent. Additionally, high blood plasma levels of ascorbic acid correlated with reduced cataract risk.

One of the problems with recommending vitamin C supplementation to prevent cataract formation is that the public is more likely to use supplements after an eye doctor diagnoses cataract. By then the hardening, discoloration, and opacification of the lens may be irreversible.

Although surgical removal of a cataract can be very effective, cataract surgery carries risks, such as increased incidence of late-stage macular dysfunction. Therefore, many research efforts focus on preventing or slowing cataract development, as well as on determining the causes of cataract formation. It is apparent that, except in those cases of cataracts that are completely congenital, the major factor in the development of this disorder is nutrient imbalance.

NUTRITIONAL SUPPLEMENTS		
Supplement	Directions for Use	Comments
Alpha-lipoic acid	200 mg daily.	Antioxidant.
Copper and manganese	2 mg copper and 10 mg manganese daily.	Slows growth of cataract.
Glutathione	As directed on label.	Antioxidant.
Grape seed extract	As directed on label.	Antioxidant.
L-lysine	As directed on label.	Important in collagen formation. Repairs the lens.
Selenium	400 mcg daily.	Antioxidant.
Superoxide dismutase (SOD)	As directed on label.	Antioxidant shown to be very effective at reducing cataract density.
Magnesium	500 mg daily.	Counteracts excessive calcium deposits.
N-acetylcarnosine (Can-C).	1 drop twice daily.	Antioxidant.
Vitamin A	3,000 IU daily.	Good for all eye conditions.
Vitamin B complex with extra B_2	75 mg vitamin B complex and 25 mg more B_2 daily.	Important for eye metabolism.
Vitamin C	2,500 mg daily.	Antioxidant.
Vitamin E	200 IU daily.	Antioxidant.
Zinc	25 mg daily. (Do not take more than 40 mg daily.)	Protects against light-induced damage.

HERBS AND HERBAL SUPPLEMENTS		
Herb	Directions for Use	Comments
Bilberry	100 mg daily. (Use extract.)	Boosts circulation. Supplies bioflavonoids.
Eyebright	Use as eyewash.	Maintains the elasticity of the lens.
Visioplex Eye Concentrate with Eyebright	As directed on label.	Promotes transfer of nutrients to the lens.

HOMEOPATHIC REMEDIES

Remedy	Directions for Use	Comments
Calcarea fluorica 6c	3 to 4 pellets under the tongue 3 to 4 times daily.	Supports connective tissue. Restores integrity of elastic fibers.
Calcarea sulfurica 6c	3 to 4 pellets under the tongue 3 to 4 times daily.	Supports connective tissue.
Causticum 6c	3 to 4 pellets under the tongue 3 to 4 times daily.	Good for elastic fibers.
Cineraria (Natural Ophthalmics)	1 to 2 drops twice daily.	Increases circulation, lymph drainage, and metabolism.
Magnesia carbonica 6c	3 to 4 pellets under the tongue 3 to 4 times daily.	Regulates acidity of bodily fluids.
Pulsatilla 6c	3 to 4 pellets under the tongue 3 to 4 times daily.	Effective during early stages of cataract formation.
Silicea 6c	3 to 4 pellets under the tongue 3 to 4 times daily.	Good for inflammation.
Sulphur 6c	3 to 4 pellets under the tongue 3 to 4 times daily.	Good for cortical cataract.

RECOMMENDATIONS

- Avoid dairy products, saturated fat, and any fat or oil that has been subjected to heat, whether during cooking or processing. These foods promote free radicals, which can damage the lens. Use cold-pressed vegetable oil only, if at all.

- Consume nine to thirteen portions of plant-based food with high antioxidant content daily. Options include spinach, broccoli, carrots, cantaloupes, and green peppers (all colorful vegetables).

- Avoid antihistamines.

- Diabetics are especially prone to cataract formation. Fortunately, purely diabetic cataracts may be reversible. Therefore, careful monitoring of blood sugar levels is critical.

- Avoid sugar, which is inflammatory.

- Wear sunglasses or a hat with a brim to reduce the effects of bright sunlight.

CENTRAL SEROUS RETINOPATHY

Central serous retinopathy (CSR) involves a collection of fluid under the macula that causes visual distortion. CSR affects adults between twenty to forty-five years of age primarily. Men are affected ten times more frequently than women. Many patients with CSR live under high levels of stress. The exact cause of CSR is controversial. Some experimental evidence suggests that high blood levels of epinephrine and other select hormones may be responsible.

Most CSR patients recover visual acuity within six months. The average recovery time is three to four months. Many patients have some residual symptoms, including distortion of shapes, color vision, contrast sensitivity, and night vision. Despite an overall good prognosis, 40 to 50 percent of patients experience one or more recurrences of this disorder.

No medical therapy has been proven effective against CSR. Laser treatment can shorten the duration of the disease but does not appear to alter final visual acuity or recurrence rate. Treatment with laser is controversial because of potential complications and lack of apparent long-term benefits. Recently, pressure patching has shown some positive results, although it should be considered only under supervision of an ophthalmologist. Nutritional therapy is designed to support retinal tissue and reduce swelling.

NUTRITIONAL SUPPLEMENTS

Supplement	Directions for Use	Comments
Longevinex	As directed on label.	Good for retinal health.
Vitamin A	3,000 IU daily.	Supports the retina.
Vitamin B complex	75 mg daily.	Good for stress.
Vitamin B6	50 to 200 mg daily.	Reduces fluid retention.
Vitamin C	2,000 to 5,000 mg daily.	Fortifies blood vessel walls.
Vitamin E	200 IU daily.	Reduces fluid retention.
Zinc	25 mg daily.	Good in combination with vitamin A.

HERBS AND HERBAL SUPPLEMENTS

Herb	Directions for Use	Comments
Alfalfa	Drink as a tea.	Good for relaxation. Good for chemical imbalance.
Chamomile	Drink as a tea.	Good for relaxation.
Gotu kola	Drink as a tea.	Good for relaxation.
Lady's slipper	Drink as a tea.	Good for relaxation.
Lobelia	Drink as a tea. (Do not take internally on an ongoing basis.)	Good for relaxation.
Passion flower	Drink as a tea.	Good for relaxation.
Valerian	Drink as a tea.	Good for relaxation.

HOMEOPATHIC REMEDIES

Remedy	Directions for Use	Comments
Apis mellifica 6c	3 to 4 pellets under the tongue 3 to 4 times daily.	Alleviates swelling.
Rhus toxicodendron 6c	3 to 4 pellets under the tongue 3 to 4 times daily.	Good for inflammation. Alleviates swelling.
Sepia 6c	3 to 4 pellets under the tongue 3 to 4 times daily.	Good for inflammation. Alleviates swelling.

RECOMMENDATIONS

- Use the Amsler Grid eye test to monitor your visual distortion.

- Practice a relaxation technique such as tai chi, yoga, or meditation.

- Practice deep, relaxed breathing.

CHALAZION

Meibomian glands are found in the rim of the eyelid. A chalazion results when one of these glands becomes obstructed. Chalazia are therefore also known as meibomian cysts and should be treated as soon as possible.

Treatment typically starts with antibiotics accompanied by hot compress-es. Chalazia occasionally grow large enough to obscure vision, at which point they need to be lanced and drained.

Nutritional support involves using omega-3 essential fatty acids in proper combination with omega-6 essential fatty acids.

NUTRITIONAL SUPPLEMENTS

Supplement	Directions for use	Comments
Omega 3 EFAs	1,000 mg daily (EPA and DHA).	Anti-inflammatory. Increases fluidity of meibomian gland secretions.
Omega-6 EFAs (Black currant seed oil)	350 mg daily.	Mucous-specific anti-inflammatory.

HERBS AND HERBAL SUPPLEMENTS

Herb	Directions for Use	Comments
Eyebright	Apply as a hot compress.	Opens pores to allow drainage.
Goldenseal	Apply as a hot compress. (Do not use during pregnancy.)	Good for eye infection.
Curcumin	500 mg daily.	Anti-inflammatory.

HOMEOPATHIC REMEDIES

Remedy	Directions for Use	Comments
Hepar sulphuris 6c	3 to 4 pellets under the tongue 3 to 4 times daily.	Good for abscesses, boils, and similar problems.
Mercurius vivus 6	3 to 4 pellets under the tongue 3 to 4 times daily.	Good for swollen glands, boils, and similar problems.
Staphysagria 6c	3 to 4 pellets under the tongue 3 to 4 times daily.	Good for extremely emotional individuals with chalazia.
Sulphur 6c	3 to 4 pellets under the tongue 3 to 4 times daily.	Good for red eyelids.
Thuja occidentalis 6c	3 to 4 pellets under the tongue 3 to 4 times daily.	Good for chalazia associated with warts.

RECOMMENDATIONS

- Do not rub your eyes with dirty hands, as doing so may lead to infection.

- Apply a warm washcloth as a compress to the affected eye as soon as possible after first noticing the chalazion. Use a compress often.

- Gently massage the chalazion lump while using a warm compress.

- Check with your eye doctor to confirm that the lump is a chalazion.

COMPUTER VISION SYNDROME

Because computer work is such a visually demanding task, it commonly results in vision problems. Most studies indicate that computer operators report more eye-related issues than do paper-oriented office workers. A study by the National Institute of Occupational Safety and Health showed 88 percent of computer users complained of computer-related eyestrain. Symptoms that typically affect computer users are now collectively known as computer vision syndrome (CVS). Symptoms may vary but usually include eyestrain, headache, blurred vision, disturbed accommodation, neck pain, light sensitivity, double vision, disturbed color vision, and dry eye.

The cause of CVS is a combination of individual visual problems, poor work habits, and poor office ergonomics. Many people have marginal vision disorders that do not cause symptoms when performing less demanding visual tasks. Working environment must be addressed in addition to visual condition when treating CVS.

Recent studies have shown that a small dose of the carotenoid astaxanthin might have an effect on visual stress due to computers. While astaxanthin is not present inside the retina, it appears to help with muscle fatigue, and thus may help with extraocular muscle stamina, eye fatigue, and other CVS symptoms.

NUTRITIONAL SUPPLEMENTS		
Supplement	Directions for Use	Comments
Astaxanthin	6 mg daily.	Helps maintain tone of striated muscle.
Vitamin A	3,000 IU daily.	Good for all eye conditions.

Supplement	Directions for Use	Commentsii
Vitamin B complex	75 mg daily.	Good for stress.
Vitamin C	3,000 mg daily.	Antioxidant. Good for stress.
Vitamin E	200 IU daily.	Antioxidant.

HERBS AND HERBAL SUPPLEMENTS		
Herb	Directions for Use	Comments
Eyebright	3 to 4 drops daily or apply as a compress.	Good for eye tissue.
Goldenseal	Apply as a compress. (Do not take internally for more than one week. Do not use during pregnancy.)	Soothes tissues.

HOMEOPATHIC REMEDIES		
Remedy	Directions for Use	Comments
Euphrasia officinalis 6c	3 to 4 pellets under the tongue 3 to 4 times daily.	Alleviates redness.
Nux vomica 6c	3 to 4 pellets under the tongue 3 to 4 times daily.	Good for eyestrain associated with overwork.
Ruta graveolens 6c	3 to 4 pellets under the tongue 3 to 4 times daily.	Good for eyestrain followed by headache. Heals tendons and ligaments.
Sulphur 6c	3 to 4 pellets under the tongue 3 to 4 times daily.	Alleviates redness following near-point work.

RECOMMENDATIONS

• Lower your monitor so when you hold your head in the normal position, you can look straight ahead and see just over the top of it.

• Make the background illumination of the screen and the illumination of your immediate work area approximately equal. You might need to dim the brightness of your screen somewhat, but don't forget to increase the contrast.

• The best screen colors to use are black letters on a white background. This combination simulates paper and ink, and provides the highest contrast between the letters and the background.

- Make sure the screen does not have any glare. To check for this, turn the computer off and look at the screen for any reflections of lights or lightly colored articles.

- Make sure there is no other light hitting your eyes, either directly from a window or lamp, or by reflection off a shiny surface.

- When working at a computer, blink often because this rests and wets the eyes.

- Breathe fully, since taking complete breaths is important in muscle relaxation.

- Take breaks from the computer. Use the "20/20/20 rule"—every twenty minutes, take twenty seconds and look twenty feet away.

CONJUNCTIVITIS

Conjunctivitis refers to inflammation of the outermost layer of the eye and inner surface of the eyelid known as the conjunctiva. It is typically caused by bacterial, viral, or fungal infection. It may also be caused by allergies or anything that has irritated the conjunctiva.

Treatment generally depends on the cause of the condition. Bacterial conjunctivitis is usually treated with hot compresses and antibiotics. Viral conjunctivitis can be treated with antivirals. Fungal forms of conjunctivitis are treated with antifungals. Allergic conjunctivitis is usually treated symptomatically—that is, by reducing itching and inflammation of eye tissue along with treating remaining allergy symptoms.

Tears contain natural antibacterial enzymes that aid in healing the eye. Nutritional support will vary with the cause of the condition and is designed to support the ocular surface as well as the tear film.

NUTRITIONAL SUPPLEMENTS		
Supplement	Directions for Use	Comments
Copper	1 mg daily.	Supports zinc use.
Omega-3 fatty acids	1,000 mg daily (EPA and DHA).	Supports the tear film.
Vitamin A	3,000 IU daily.	Good for epithelial cell support.

Supplement	Directions for Use	Comments
Vitamin C	2,000 to 6,000 mg in divided doses daily.	Supports tissue healing and the tear film.
Zinc	25 mg daily.	Enhances immune response.

HERBS AND HERBAL SUPPLEMENTS		
Herb	Directions for Use	Comments
Chamomile	Apply as a hot compress or use as an eyewash.	Soothes eye tissue.
Eyebright and fennel	Apply as a hot compress or use as an eyewash.	Boosts circulation.

HOMEOPATHIC REMEDIES		
Remedy	Directions for Use	Comments
Aconite 6c	3 to 4 pellets under the tongue 3 to 4 times daily.	Good for inflammation.
Allium cepa 6c	3 to 4 pellets under the tongue.	Good for inflammation.
Anacardium 6c	3 to 4 pellets under the tongue.	Alleviates swelling.
Apis mellifica 6c	3 to 4 pellets under the tongue.	Good for pinkeye with swollen eyelids. Alleviates edema and inflammation.
Arnica montana 6c	3 to 4 pellets under the tongue.	Good for inflammation.
Arsenicum album 6c	3 to 4 pellets under the tongue.	Good for inflammation.
Belladonna 6c	3 to 4 pellets under the tongue.	Good for inflammation.
Calcarea fluorica 6c	3 to 4 pellets under the tongue 3 to 4 times daily.	Relieves discharge. Good for inflammation.
Calcarea sulfurica 6c	3 to 4 pellets under the tongue 3 to 4 times daily.	Relieves discharge. Good for inflammation.
Causticum 6c	3–4 pellets under the tongue.	Relieves discharge.

Remedy	Directions for Use	Comments
Euphrasia officinalis 6c	3 to 4 pellets under the tongue 3 to 4 times daily.	Good for inflammation.
Graphites 9c	3 to 4 pellets under the tongue 3 to 4 times daily.	Good for inflamed eyelids.
Mercurius corrosivus 6c	3 to 4 pellets under the tongue 3 to 4 times daily.	Good for pinkeye with mucous discharge. Fights infection.
Mercurius vivus 6c	3 to 4 pellets under the tongue 3 to 4 times daily.	Relieves discharge. Good for inflammation.
Natrum muriaticum 6c	3 to 4 pellets under the tongue 3 to 4 times daily.	Good for inflammation.
Pulsatilla 6c	3 to 4 pellets under the tongue 3 to 4 times daily.	Relieves discharge. Good for inflammation and allergic conjunctivitis.
Rhus toxicodendron 6c	3 to 4 pellets under the tongue 3 to 4 times daily.	Good for inflammation. Alleviates swelling.
Ruta graveolens 6c	3 to 4 pellets under the tongue 3 to 4 times daily.	Good for inflammation.
Sepia 6c	3 to 4 pellets under the tongue 3 to 4 times daily.	Good for inflammation. Alleviates swelling.
Silicea 6c	3 to 4 pellets under the tongue 3 to 4 times daily.	Good for inflammation.
Sulphur 6c	3 to 4 pellets under the tongue 3 to 4 times daily.	Good for inflammation and allergic conjunctivitis.

RECOMMENDATIONS

- Conjunctivitis is one of the most contagious diseases currently known. Children seem to be more susceptible to it, probably due to their lack of proper hygiene. Children should be taught to wash their hands properly and to keep their hands away from their eyes.

- It is also very helpful to wash out your eyes with cold water if you've been around something to which you're allergic. Do not use an "eye-cup," as it will harbor the allergen and may cause the problem to recur.

- If itchiness is a symptom, do not use any over-the-counter preparations that promise to remove redness from the eyes.

- Conjunctivitis may be treated with a hot compress two to three times a day, specifically if the eyelids are sticking together in the morning.

CORNEAL ABRASION

Corneal abrasion is any disruption on the surface of the cornea. A foreign body or scratch on the cornea is typically the cause of this condition. Oftentimes, the foreign body is no longer present but the patient feels some discomfort when the eyelid passes over the abraded area.

Most corneal abrasions heal within a few days, although certain injuries may take longer than others. Caution should be taken to assure the wound is clean. Nutritional support is directed towards healing the wound and strengthening the corneal tissue.

NUTRITIONAL SUPPLEMENTS

Supplement	Directions for Use	Comments
Omega-3 essential fatty acids	1,000 mg daily (EPA and DHA).	Supports the tear film.
Vitamin A drops (Retinoic acid)	1 to 2 drops 3 to 4 times daily for two days.	Supports the corneal tissue as it heals.
Vitamin C	500 mg twice daily for two days.	Builds collagen tissue.
Vitamin B2	75 mg daily.	Helps collagen crosslinking.

HERBS AND HERBAL SUPPLEMENTS

Herb	Directions for Use	Comments
Bayberry, eyebright, and goldenseal	Use as an eyewash twice daily. (Do not take internally for more than one week. Do not use during pregnancy.)	Good for all eye conditions.
Comfrey	Use as an eyewash.	Promotes healing.
White willow bark	400 mg as needed.	Good for pain.

HOMEOPATHIC REMEDIES

Remedy	Directions for Use	Comments
Aconite 6c	3 to 4 pellets under the tongue 3 to 4 times daily.	Good for general eye discomfort.

Remedy	Directions for Use	Comments
Aurum 6c	3 to 4 pellets under the tongue 3 to 4 times daily.	Good for pain.
Belladonna 6c	3 to 4 pellets under the tongue 3 to 4 times daily.	Good for pain.
Bryonia 6c	3 to 4 pellets under the tongue 3 to 4 times daily.	Good for pain.
Chamomilla 6c	3 to 4 pellets under the tongue 3 to 4 times daily.	Good for pain.
Cinchona officinalis 6c	3 to 4 pellets under the tongue 3 to 4 times daily.	Good for pain.
Hypericum perforatum 6c	3 to 4 pellets under the tongue 3 to 4 times daily.	Good for nerve injury.
Lycopodium 6c	3 to 4 pellets under the tongue 3 to 4 times daily.	Good for pain.
Mercurius vivus 6c	3 to 4 pellets under the tongue 3 to 4 times daily.	Good for corneal abrasions accompanied by discharge.
Natrum muriaticum 6c	3 to 4 pellets under the tongue 3 to 4 times daily.	Good for pain.
Nitricum acidum 6c	3 to 4 pellets under the tongue 3 to 4 times daily.	Good for pain.
Sanguinaria 6c	3 to 4 pellets under the tongue 3 to 4 times daily.	Good for pain.
Staphysagria 6c	3 to 4 pellets under the tongue 3 to 4 times daily.	Good for corneal abrasions associated with anger.
Spigelia 6c	3 to 4 pellets under the tongue 3 to 4 times daily.	Good for pain.

RECOMMENDATIONS

- Get plenty of rest.

- Take an over-the-counter pain medication if homeopathic remedies aren't effective.

- Use a cool compress to reduce inflammation.

- If your eye doesn't feel normal again in twenty-four to thirty-six hours, see your eye doctor.

CORNEAL ULCER

The cause of most corneal ulcers today is related to contact lens wearing. The lens being in constant contact with the corneal surface, combined with poor lens hygiene or extended usage can lead to a break in the corneal surface and an opening for bacteria to invade. Corneal ulcers require a rapid response with proper medical treatment. Nutritional support is important in the healing process, and patients should seriously consider lifestyle changes to aid in resolving this condition and preventing recurrence.

NUTRITIONAL SUPPLEMENTS

Supplement	Directions for Use	Comments
Folic acid	5 mg 3 times daily.	Aids in tissue healing.
Vitamin A	3,000 IU daily.	Good for epithelial cell health.
Vitamin B_2	100 mg daily.	Aids in nerve healing.
Vitamin C	4,000 mg divided doses throughout the day.	Aids in tissue healing.
Vitamin E	200 IU daily.	Aids in tissue healing.
Omega-3 essential fatty acids	1,000 to 3,000 mg daily (EPA and DHA).	Anti-inflammatory. Supports anterior ocular surface.

HERBS AND HERBAL SUPPLEMENTS

Herb	Directions for Use	Comments
Eyebright	1 to 2 drops 4 to 5 times daily.	Good for overall eye healing. Begin taking after you have finished taking other drops.

HOMEOPATHIC REMEDIES

Remedy	Directions for Use	Comments
Aconite 6c	3 to 4 pellets under the tongue 3 to 4 times daily.	Alleviates pain and inflammation in early stages of corneal ulcer formation.
Apis mellifica 6c	3 to 4 pellets under the tongue 3 to 4 times daily.	Good for inflammation.

Remedy	Directions for Use	Comments
Calcarea sulfurica 6c	3 to 4 pellets under the tongue 3 to 4 times daily.	Reduces light sensitivity.
Euphrasia officinalis 6c	3 to 4 pellets under the tongue 3 to 4 times daily.	Good for all eye conditions.
Mercurius corrosivus 6c	3 to 4 pellets under the tongue 3 to 4 times daily.	Good for pain.

RECOMMENDATIONS

- If you experience any sharp pain or discomfort around the eyes, see your eye doctor immediately.

- If you wear contact lenses and feel discomfort, remove them immediately and do not use them again until your eyes feel comfortable. If your eyes continue to feel uncomfortable, see your doctor.

- Ulcers can cause permanent vision loss if they are not dealt with quickly and effectively, so pay attention to your doctor's instructions.

- Keep excessive makeup away from the area, and be sure not to touch the area with unwashed fingers.

DIABETIC RETINOPATHY

The global prevalence of diabetes has been increasing and is projected to rise to 366 million people by 2030, a 39-percent increase since 2000. Unless this trend is reversed, the number of people afflicted with diabetic retinopathy is likely to climb as well. Currently, laser therapy is the primary means of treating diabetic retinopathy and can reduce the progression of the condition. Without treatment, this problem only worsens. A long-term epidemiological study in the United States found this rate of progression of diabetic retinopathy of 86 percent over a fourteen-year follow-up.

In theory, antioxidants may treat this condition by retarding oxidative damage to the retina, but there are no relevant clinical studies of antioxidants and diabetic retinopathy at this time. Some studies have suggested a link between the microvascular damage associated with retinopathy and elevated homocysteine levels. In general, reducing the overall physical effects of diabetes will alter the retinal ramifications of the disease process.

If treated properly through lifestyle changes, the disease process may actually reverse, possibly saving the vision of the individual.

At the onset of diabetes, before blood sugar is brought under control, diabetics often experience blurred vision. This is because high blood sugar causes fluid retention changes in the crystalline lens. Blurred vision may, in fact, be the first sign of diabetes. After the proper insulin dosage is determined and the disease is stabilized, the blurred vision resolves, although it may recur if blood sugar rises again. Diabetic retinopathy typically occurs about ten to twelve years into the disorder, but sometimes sooner. If left unchecked, retinal hemorrhages and fluid leaks will eventually spill into the vitreous, where they may scar and pull on the retina, often causing retinal detachment and blindness.

Of course, the best treatment for diabetes is to prevent it from happening in the first place. There is evidence that staying in good diabetic control—that is, keeping blood sugar levels normal through diet and insulin—minimizes long-term as well as short-term complications of the disorder. There is also a slight hereditary factor, so if you have a parent with diabetes, your risk is elevated and you should be especially careful to eat a healthy diet and get regular medical checkups. Environmental factors, however, tend to play more of a role in the development of diabetes than do genetic factors.

NUTRITIONAL SUPPLEMENTS		
Supplement	Directions for Use	Comments
Alpha-lipoic acid	200 mg daily.	Improves blood sugar control.
Chromium picolinate	400 to 600 mcg daily.	Improves insulin efficiency.
Longevinex	As directed on label.	Supports retinal structures.
Magnesium	500 mg daily.	Protects against arterial spasm.
Manganese	2 mg daily.	Enzyme activator.
Niacin	20 mg daily.	Small amounts increase circulation.
Potassium	300 mg daily.	Maintains proper fluid balance.
Selenium	100 mcg daily.	Suppresses development of new blood vessels.

Supplement	Directions for Use	Comments
Vitamin A	3,000 IU daily.	Recommended for diabetics, who often have difficulty converting beta-carotene into vitamin A.
Vitamin B-complex	75 mg daily.	Boosts circulation.
Vitamin C with bioflavonoids	1,000 mg evenly divided daily. (Use powdered buffered ascorbic acid.)	Reduces the chance of vascular problems developing.
Vitamin D$_3$	5,000 IU daily.	Supports the immune system.
Vitamin E	200 IU daily.	Aids in tissue healing. Antioxidant.

HERBS AND HERBAL SUPPLEMENTS

Herb	Directions for Use	Comments
Cinnamon	Up to 6 g daily.	Improves glucose and lipid metabolism in diabetics.
Comfrey	Drink as a tea.	Strengthens blood.
Dandelion	Drink as a tea.	Boosts activity of the pancreas.
Ginseng	Drink as a tea.	Normalizes blood.
Gymnema sylvestre	Drink as a tea.	Helps the pancreas produce insulin.
Yarrow	Drink as a tea.	Controls bleeding.

HOMEOPATHIC REMEDIES

Remedy	Directions for Use	Comments
Lachesis 6c	3 to 4 pellets under the tongue 3 to 4 times daily.	Restores vascular integrity.
Natrum sulfuricum 6c	3 to 4 pellets under the tongue 3 to 4 times daily.	Supports pancreatic function.
Phosphorus 6c	3 to 4 pellets under the tongue 3 to 4 times daily.	Improves metabolism of vascular tissue.
Syzygium jambolanum 6c	3 to 4 pellets under the tongue 3 to 4 times daily.	Supports glucose metabolism.
Uranium nitricum 6c	3 to 4 pellets under the tongue 3 to 4 times daily.	Stabilizes glucose levels.

RECOMMENDATIONS

- Since diabetes is a systemic disease, even control of diabetic eye changes is initially done using general treatments such as diet and exercise.

- Have your blood sugar level checked regularly, especially if diabetes runs in your family.

- If you notice any fluctuations in your vision, request that you be tested for diabetes.

- Once you are diagnosed with diabetic retinopathy, you should have a dilated eye exam once a year, and more often if recommended by your doctor.

DRY EYE SYNDROME

Dry eye syndrome is a problem with either the quantity or quality of the tear film of the eye, leading to symptoms that include dryness, redness, burning, grittiness, and excessive tearing. At one time, dry eye syndrome was not considered a disease but rather a group of symptoms associated with conditions such as allergies or arthritis, the use of certain medication, and environmental factors such as low humidity and computer use. We now know it is a specific disease process (an inflammation) that may be exaggerated by these conditions. Traditional dry eye treatment involves medication in the form of artificial tears or pharmaceutical solutions used to restore tear production.

Chronic dry eye syndrome may be the result of an accumulation of free radicals in tissue due to age, stress (including the stress of corneal surgery or contact lens wear), or general degeneration. Studies point to nutritional deficiency as a major contributor to the accumulation of free radicals in the lacrimal, mucous, and oil-producing glands of the eye. Research shows that specifically targeted nutritional supplements can restore function to these glands and provide lubrication to the eye. Certain antioxidants, in particular, may restore and support tear function. Essential fatty acids have also shown promise in the treatment of dry eye syndrome. Some practitioners are still using flax oil as treatment for dry eye syndrome because it contains a large amount of omega-3s and a small amount of omega-6s. Unfortunately, flax oil is highly unstable and contains none of the nutrient cofactors necessary to ensure resolution of the problem. Pharmaceutical-grade cod liver oil as a source of omega-3s is one of the most effective formulations. It serves as an excellent source of vitamins A and D, which are both necessary for a healthy base layer of the tear film.

A combination of vitamin C, vitamin B_6, and magnesium promotes cellular defense against invading pathogens and allergens, which frequently cause dry eye symptoms. Green tea may also fight against dry eye syndrome thanks to its rich content of antioxidant compounds such as epigallocatechin gallate (EGCG) and catechins. Catechins scavenge for free radicals and EGCG seems to protect retinal ganglion cells against oxidative injury.

NUTRITIONAL SUPPLEMENTS

Supplement	Directions for Use	Comments
BioTears (Biosyntrx)	As directed on label.	Supports healthy tears.
Coenzyme Q_{10}	80 mg daily.	Antioxidant.
Black currant seed oil	1,000 mg at bedtime daily.	Supplies essential fatty acids.
Iodine	75 mcg daily.	Supports healthy tear glands.
Vitamin A	3,000 IU daily.	Supports corneal epithelial cells.
Vitamin B_6	50 mg daily.	Regulates kidney function.
Vitamin C	7,500 mg evenly divided throughout the day.	Antioxidant.

HERBS AND HERBAL SUPPLEMENTS

Herb	Directions for Use	Comments
Chamomile	Use warm as an infusion. Use cool as an eyewash.	Supports eye tissue.
Green Tea	4 to 6 cups a day.	Antioxidant.
Goldenseal	Use warm as an infusion. Use cool as an eyewash. (Do not use during pregnancy.)	Supports eye tissue.

HOMEOPATHIC REMEDIES

Remedy	Directions for Use	Comments
Aconite 6c	3 to 4 pellets under the tongue 3 to 4 times daily.	Alleviates dryness.
Alumina 6c	3 to 4 pellets under the tongue 3 to 4 times daily.	Alleviates dryness.
Arsenicum album 6c	3 to 4 pellets under the tongue 3 to 4 times daily.	Alleviates dryness.
Belladonna 6c	3 to 4 pellets under the tongue 3 to 4 times daily.	Good for dry eye associated with fever and redness.
Dry Eye Formula (Natural Ophthalmics)	1 to 2 drops daily as needed for relief.	Two different formulas exist: One for men and one for women.
Euphrasia officinalis 6c	3 to 4 pellets under the tongue 3 to 4 times daily.	Good for dry eye associated with wind.
Optique 1 (Boiron)	1 to 2 drops daily as needed for relief.	A good general remedy.
Pulsatilla 6c	3 to 4 pellets under the tongue 3 to 4 times daily.	Alleviates dryness.
Similisan No. 1	1 to 2 drops daily as needed for relief.	Good for red, dry eyes.
Sulphur 6c	3 to 4 pellets under the tongue 3 to 4 times daily.	Alleviates dryness. Reduces redness.
Veratrum album 6c	3 to 4 pellets under the tongue 3 to 4 times daily.	Alleviates dryness.
Zincum metallicum 6c	3 to 4 pellets under the tongue 3 to 4 times daily.	Alleviates dryness.

RECOMMENDATIONS

- Use preservative-free eye drops for lubrication.

- If you have dry eyes, contact your eye doctor before changing your diet. In addition to your specific eye condition, medical history, prescription medication, and allergies all need to be taken into account.

- Use humidifiers in your home. This is especially important if you live in a dry area or at high altitude.

- Wear wraparound sun goggles outdoors. Sunglasses (or even clear goggles) with side shields can help to reduce the evaporation of moisture from the eye by as much as 40 percent.

- Blink! When you blink, you squeeze out tears from glands in your eyelids. Waiting twenty to thirty seconds between blinks may cause the tear film to break, which can lead to dehydration of the surface of the eye. We normally blink about twenty times a minute.

- Quit smoking. Cigarette smoke causes dry spots to develop on the surface of the eye 40-percent faster than when the lids are held open.

- Avoid smog and fumes. Smog and fumes not only cause dry and irritated eyes, they also inactivate the enzyme that acts as an antibacterial agent in the tear fluid.

- If you use a computer, place the monitor so that your eyes aim downward when you look at it. This will allow you to keep your eyes partially closed, reducing the surface area of the eye exposed to air.

- Reduce, replace, or avoid eye makeup. Eye makeup has been shown to thin the oily layer of the tear film, which keeps the eye from becoming dehydrated. It can harbor bacteria and should be replaced frequently. Gentle removal of all eye makeup every night is essential.

- Check your medication. Some medications can cause dry eyes as a side effect. These medications include antihistamines, atropine, beta blockers, cancer medications, codeine, decongestant eye drops, decongestants, morphine, allergy medications, scopolamine, tranquilizers, and vitamin-A analogs. The artificial sweetener aspartame, excessive supplemental vitamin B_3, and the recreational drug hashish can also cause dry eye.

- Check your soft contact lenses. Soft contact lenses often promote the evaporation of tears from the surface of the eye. In severe dry eye cases, contact lenses cannot be worn.

GIANT PAPILLARY CONJUNCTIVITIS

Giant papillary conjunctivitis (GPC) is a type of ocular inflammatory reaction that usually occurs in soft contact lens wearers. It is a chronic low grade allergic reaction in the conjunctiva of the upper lid. This disorder can also develop over time from irritation caused by a surgical suture or other foreign body. While it is much more uncommon these days (due to improved contact lens materials and flexible wearing schedules), it can still be an issue for those who are sensitive and do not take proper care of their lenses.

In most cases, treatment of GPC involves discontinuing the use of contact lenses to allow the eye to recover on its own. Contacts may need to be avoided for several days or weeks. Severe cases may take even longer to resolve.

NUTRITIONAL SUPPLEMENTS

Supplement	Directions for Use	Comments
Copper	1 mg daily.	Needed with zinc supplementation.
Fish oil	1,500 mg daily (EPA and DHA).	Maintains moisture in mucous membranes.
Vitamin A	3,000 IU daily.	Maintains moisture in the eye.
Vitamin B complex	50 to 100 mg daily.	Improves intraocular cellular metabolism.
Vitamin C	2,000 to 6,000 mg daily.	Protects the eye from further inflammation.
Zinc	25 mg daily.	Enhances immune response.

HERBS AND HERBAL SUPPLEMENTS

Herb	Directions for Use	Comments
Eyebright	Use as an eyewash.	Good for all eye conditions.
Goldenseal	Apply as a compress. (Do not use during pregnancy.)	Soothes mucous membranes.

HOMEOPATHIC REMEDIES		
Remedy	**Directions for Use**	**Comments**
Allium cepa 6c	3 to 4 pellets under the tongue 3 to 4 times daily.	Relieves mucous discharge.
Apis mellifica 6c	3 to 4 pellets under the tongue 3 to 4 times daily.	Alleviates swelling.
Mercurius corrosivus 6c	3 to 4 pellets under the tongue 3 to 4 times daily.	Relieves mucous discharge.
Pulsatilla 6c	3 to 4 pellets under the tongue 3 to 4 times daily.	Relieves mucous discharge.

RECOMMENDATIONS

- Change your contact lenses often. Fresh lenses cause GPC far less than older soiled lenses do.

- Switch to a different type of lens. Eyes with GPC often tolerate daily disposable soft lenses (thrown away every night). Some lens materials aggravate GPC more than others.

- Wear your lenses only occasionally. Change the soaking solution every week if lenses are not worn.

- A cold compress used several times a day will help to relieve itching associated with GPC.

- Since GPC is a form of pinkeye, the same treatments and recommendations associated with that condition are effective in connection with GPC.

GLAUCOMA

Glaucoma is a condition in which intraocular pressure is markedly elevated. This increase prevents blood from reaching, nourishing, and circulating through the eye. If the pressure remains high for an extended period of time, it causes death of the optic nerve. Worldwide, glaucoma is second only to cataract as a leading cause of blindness. Most sufferers have few or no symptoms of the disease, which occurs in 1 to 2 percent of the over-forty population and is a common cause of blindness in the United States. A family history of glaucoma or diabetes, previous eye injury or surgery, and use of ocular steroids are considered risk factors for developing glaucoma.

Studies of nutraceutical antioxidants, including ginkgo biloba, bilberry, red sage, and lipoic acid, have met with modest success in improving visual acuity and peripheral vision in people with glaucoma, possibly by improving circulation to the optic nerve. Elevated levels of homocysteine and depressed levels of folate (but not vitamin B_{12}) were correlated with pseudoexfoliative glaucoma in one study. Another study found vitamin B_{12} supplementation to be beneficial in glaucoma treatment. A small study of DHA supplementation in the elderly found improvements in visual acuity in some subjects with cataract and glaucoma. In summary, research on the role of nutrients and glaucoma is suggestive but still very preliminary.

Over the past few years, a combination or Pycnogenol and bilberry extract has displayed a pressure-lowering effect in a number of studies. This formula, known as Mirtogenol, may lower eye pressure slightly and increase blood delivery to the optic nerve. Studies also suggest that the coupling of Mirtogenol with an existing glaucoma medication may result in better outcomes than either of the two treatments alone.

According to one theory of glaucoma development, prolonged stress and inadequate diet over a long period of time are considered to be primary causative factors. Prolonged stress leads to adrenal exhaustion, and exhausted adrenal glands are no longer able to produce aldosterone, which stabilizes the body's salt balance. When too much salt is lost from the body, tissue fluids build up and often will push into the eyeball, increasing intraocular pressure and damaging the optic nerve.

Much has been made in recent years of the use of marijuana to treat glaucoma. While there has been some research on this option, the studies are not definitive. One effect of marijuana is a lowering of intraocular pressure, though the mechanism of action is still not known. Therefore, it does reduce eye pressure, albeit for a short period of time (about three to four hours). There are many other medications, of course, that achieve this desired effect more easily and with less of a euphoric side effect.

Since one cause of glaucoma may be adrenal exhaustion, as discussed above, it is important to give adrenal glands nutritional support. Many of these supplements should be taken along with any medication prescribed. Exercise also seems effective at reducing eye pressure, but be sure to check with your doctor before starting any exercise program.

NUTRITIONAL SUPPLEMENTS		
Supplement	**Directions for Use**	**Comments**
Black currant seed oil	50 mg daily.	Antioxidant.
Choline and inositol	1,000 to 2,000 mg of a combination supplement daily.	Support eye health.
Fish oil	2,000 mg daily (EPA and DHA).	Has been shown to lower eye pressure.
Glutathione	500 mg twice daily.	Antioxidant.
Longevinex	As directed on label.	Anti-inflammatory.
Manganese	4 mg daily.	Enzyme activator.
Mirtogenol	1 pill in the morning and 1 pill in the evening.	Increases ocular perfusion.
Rutin	50 mg 3 times daily.	Works with vitamin C to reduce eye pressure.
Vitamin A	3,000 IU daily.	Aids in the metabolism of certain molecules in mucous.
Vitamin B_5	100 mg 3 times daily.	Supports health of adrenal glands.
Vitamin C	2,000 mg spread out evenly throughout the day.	Reduces eye pressure.
Vitamin E	200 IU daily.	Increases blood flow to posterior ciliary arteries.

HERBS AND HERBAL SUPPLEMENTS		
Herb	**Directions for Use**	**Comments**
Bilberry	As directed on label.	Antioxidant.
Eyebright	Drink as a tea.	Good for all eye conditions.
Ginkgo biloba and zinc sulfate	As directed on label.	Increases circulation.
Rose hips	Drink as a tea.	A source of vitamin C.

HOMEOPATHIC REMEDIES

Remedy	Directions for Use	Comments
Belladonna 6c	3 to 4 pellets under the tongue 3 to 4 times daily.	Relieves colored halo around lights.
Nux vomica 6c	3 to 4 pellets under the tongue 3 to 4 times daily.	Good for high eye pressure.
Phosphorus 6c	3 to 4 pellets under the tongue 3 to 4 times daily.	Relieves colored halo around lights.
Pulsatilla 6c	3 to 4 pellets under the tongue 3 to 4 times daily.	Relieves colored halo around lights.
Sulphur 6c	3 to 4 pellets under the tongue 3 to 4 times daily.	Good for glaucoma associated with pain.

RECOMMENDATIONS

- It is critical to have your eye pressure checked regularly to monitor the progress of your glaucoma.

- Since peripheral vision is affected first, be sure to have it tested periodically.

- Be careful when drinking large amounts of fluid. Moderate amounts are recommended.

- Avoid tobacco smoke, nicotine, alcohol, and caffeine.

- Avoid refined carbohydrates, such as white bread, which are taxing to the adrenal glands.

- A diet consisting of a higher omega-6 to omega-3 fat intake may offer some protection against developing glaucoma.

GRAVE'S DISEASE

Grave's disease is one of the more common types of hyperthyroidism. It is a disorder in which the thyroid gland produces too much thyroid hormone, resulting in an overactive metabolism. As the body's processes speed up, symptoms may include nervousness, irritability, a constant feeling of being hot, increased perspiration, excessive tearing, dry eye, insomnia, and fatigue. Patients may also present symptoms of goiter, exophthalmos, tachycardia, weight loss, hyperactive reflexes, drooping eyelids, and tremor. The size of the thyroid gland may be normal in a small number of patients. Eye symptoms may include pain, excessive tearing, blurred vision, double vision, lid retraction (which creates the appearance of bulging eyes), swelling, optic nerve inflammation, and enlargement of extraocular muscles. The age of onset of Grave's disease is most commonly between thirty and forty years old. Females are affected seven times more often than men.

Because Grave's disease is a metabolic disturbance, it is imperative that patients watch their diets closely. While hyperthyroidism can't be treated through diet alone, if you are diagnosed with this issue, be sure to eat *Brassica* vegetables, which help to suppress the production of thyroid hormone. These include broccoli, cauliflower, kale, and cabbage. Your diet should also contain berries, which are powerful antioxidants that help to support the immune system. In addition, protein is important for energy and maintenance of muscle, which can be lost as a result of Grave's disease. Calcium intake is also crucial to support maintenance of bones.

NUTRITIONAL SUPPLEMENTS		
Supplement	**Directions for Use**	**Comments**
BioTears (Biosyntrx)	As directed on label.	Maintains eye moisture.
Fish oil	3,000 mg daily (EPA and DHA).	Increases tear retention.
GLA	300 mg with each meal.	Maintains eye moisture.
Glutamine	2 g upon waking.	Supports mucous tissue.
Magnesium	400 to 800 mg.	Slow release may be needed.
Multivitamin	As directed on label.	People with Grave's disease need increased amounts of all vitamins and minerals.
Vitamin B complex	50 mg 3 times daily with meals.	Benefits thyroid function.
Vitamin B$_1$	Take 50 mg twice daily.	Benefits blood formation and energy levels.

Supplement	Directions for Use	Comments
Vitamin B$_2$	Take 50 mg twice daily.	Supports functions of all cells, glands, and organs.
Vitamin B$_6$	Take 50 mg twice daily.	Enzyme activator. Necessary for proper immune function and antibody production.
Vitamin C	500 mg 3 times daily.	Antioxidant.
Vitamin E	200 IU daily.	Antioxidant.

HERBS AND HERBAL SUPPLEMENTS

Herb	Directions for Use	Comments
Alfalfa	As directed on label.	Good source of vitamin K. Good for relaxation.
Burdock	As directed on label.	Good source of iron.
Eyebright	Use as an eyewash.	Maintains eye moisture.
Gotu kola	As directed on label.	Good for relaxation.
Kelp	As directed on label.	Fights infection.
Licorice	As directed on label.	Good for stress.

HOMEOPATHIC REMEDIES

Remedy	Directions for Use	Comments
Aconite 6c	3 to 4 pellets under the tongue 3 to 4 times daily.	Good for anxiety.
Arsenicum album 6c	3 to 4 pellets under the tongue 3 to 4 times daily.	Good for anxiety.
Belladonna 6c	3 to 4 pellets under the tongue 3 to 4 times daily.	Good for restlessness.
Iodium 6c	3 to 4 pellets under the tongue 3 to 4 times daily.	Restores iodine intake by the thyroid gland.
Thyroidium 6c	3 to 4 pellets under the tongue 3 to 4 times daily.	Regulates metabolism.

RECOMMENDATIONS

- Avoid dairy products for at least three months. Also avoid stimulants, including coffee, tea, nicotine, and soft drinks.

- Be aware of the possible side effects of treatment with radioactive sodium iodine, which include hypersensitivity, radiation toxicity, and metabolic events. Talk to your doctor extensively about these matters before opting for surgery.

- To help with your eye symptoms, use eyewashes and artificial tears to maintain eye moisture.

HEADACHE

A headache, or cephalalgia, is pain anywhere in the region of the head or neck. It is one of the most common reasons patients seek an appointment with their eyecare provider. It can be a symptom of a number of different conditions of the head and neck. Brain tissue itself is not sensitive to pain because it lacks pain receptors. Rather, headache pain is caused by a disturbance of pain-sensitive structures around the brain. Nine areas of the head and neck have these pain-sensitive structures. These areas are the cranium, muscles, nerves, arteries and veins, subcutaneous tissue, eyes, ears, sinuses, and mucous membranes.

There are a number of different classification systems for headaches. The most recognized is that of the International Headache Society. Treatment of this condition depends on the underlying cause, but commonly involves analgesics. It is very often the first sign of a vision-related problem, though almost everyone experiences headache at one time or another. Common causes are stress, tension, anxiety, allergies, constipation, coffee consumption, hunger, sinus pressure, muscular tension, hormone imbalance, trauma, nutritional deficiency, alcohol consumption, drug use, smoking, fever, and eyestrain.

Experts estimate that about 90 percent of all headaches are tension headaches and 6 percent are migraines. Tension headaches, as the name implies, are caused by muscular tension. Migraines result from, most likely, a disturbance in blood circulation to the brain. Another type of headache is the cluster headache. This is a severe, recurring headache that strikes one to two individuals per thousand people.

There are many options for treating a headache. Most of them involve discovering the condition that led to the headache and then treating that condition. People who suffer from frequent headaches may be reacting to certain foods or food additives such as wheat, chocolate, monosodium glutamate (MSG), sulfites, sugar, fermented foods (such as cheese, sour cream, and yogurt), alcohol, vinegar, or marinated foods. Other possible causes include anemia, bowel problems, brain disorders, teeth grinding, high blood pressure, low blood sugar, sinusitis, spinal misalignment, overdose of vitamin A, deficiency of vitamin B, and certain eye disorders.

NUTRITIONAL SUPPLEMENTS

Supplement	Directions for Use	Comments
Bromelain	500 mg as needed.	Helps to regulate inflammatory response.
Calcium	1,500 mg daily.	Relieves muscular tension.
Coenzyme Q_{10}	30 mg twice daily.	Improves tissue oxygenation.
Glucosamine sulfate	As directed on label.	A natural alternative to aspirin and NSAIDs.
Magnesium	1,000 mg daily.	Relieves muscular tension.
Potassium	100 mg daily.	Maintains proper balance between sodium and potassium.
Vitamin B complex	50 mg 3 times daily.	Good for nerve function.
Vitamin C	2,000 to 8,000 mg in divided doses daily.	Antioxidant. Good for stress.
Vitamin E	200 IU daily.	Boosts circulation.

HERBS AND HERBAL SUPPLEMENTS

Herb	Directions for Use	Comments
Burdock	As directed on label.	Excellent detoxifier.
Evening primrose oil	500 mg 3 to 4 times daily.	Supplies essential fatty acids, which promote circulation.
Fenugreek	As directed on label.	Good for headache.
Feverfew	As directed on label. (Do not use during pregnancy.)	Good for headache.

Herb	Directions for Use	Comments
Goldenseal	As directed on label. (Do not take internally for more than one week. Do not use during pregnancy.)	Soothes tissues.
Lavender	Rub essential oil on temples.	Good for headache accompanied by stomach upset.
Lobelia	As directed on label. (Do not take internally.)	Good for tension headache.
Marshmallow	As directed on label.	Anti-inflammatory.
Mint	Rub essential oil on sore area.	Calms nerves.
Rosemary	As directed on label.	Boosts circulation.
Skullcap	As directed on label.	Relieves spasm.
Thyme	As directed on label.	Good for sinus headache.
White willow bark	As directed on label.	Good for pain.

HOMEOPATHIC REMEDIES

Remedy	Directions for Use	Comments
Aconite 6c	3 to 4 pellets under the tongue 3 to 4 times daily.	Good for throbbing headache.
Arsenicum album 6c	3 to 4 pellets under the tongue 3 to 4 times daily.	Good for head colds.
Belladonna 6c	3 to 4 pellets under the tongue 3 to 4 times daily.	Good for cold, flu, sore throat, and similar problems.
Bryonia 6c	3 to 4 pellets under the tongue 3 to 4 times daily.	Relieves pressure inside head.
Gelsemium sempervirens 6c	3 to 4 pellets under the tongue 3 to 4 times daily.	Good for headache that forms a band around the head.
Nux vomica 6c	3 to 4 pellets under the tongue 3 to 4 times daily.	Good for headache at back of head or over eyes. Good for sharp pain and eyestrain resulting from overwork.
Ruta graveolens 6c	3 to 4 pellets under the tongue 3 to 4 times daily.	Supports tendons and ligaments.
Sulphur 6c	3 to 4 pellets under the tongue 3 to 4 times daily.	Relieves burning sensation at top of the head.

RECOMMENDATIONS

- Eat a well-balanced diet. Avoid bubble gum, ice cream, iced beverages, and salt.

- Avoid excessive sunlight directed at the eyes.

- Practice deep-breathing exercises. A lack of oxygen can cause headache.

- If you use a computer, take breaks often. (See Computer Vision Syndrome on page 69.)

- Always seek and treat the cause of a headache. Long-term reliance on aspirin or other painkillers can make chronic headaches worse by interfering with the brain's natural ability to fight them.

- Many times, lying down and remaining quiet for a short period of time will alleviate a headache, especially a tension headache. You might also try a cold washcloth over the painful spot to reduce excessive blood flow to the area.

- Caffeine can work to reduce headache pain because it constricts blood vessels, although it is less effective if you are a regular coffee drinker.

HYPERTENSIVE RETINOPATHY

Hypertensive retinopathy is a pathological condition of the retina directly caused by hypertension, or high blood pressure. Because many of the blood vessels of the eye lie within the structure of the retina, any condition that affects blood vessels may, in turn, affect the retina. It is beyond the scope of this book to discuss the causes of hypertension, but it is certainly worth looking at how to control the disorder with lifestyle modifications. High blood pressure most often has no symptoms. Warning signs associated with advanced hypertension include headache, sweating, rapid pulse, shortness of breath, dizziness, and visual disturbances.

Hypertension comprises two forms of high blood pressure: primary and secondary. Primary hypertension is associated with smoking, stress, obesity, stimulant intake, drug abuse, high sodium intake, and oral contraceptive use. Secondary hypertension occurs when blood pressure rises as a result of another health problem. It may also result from blood vessels being chronically constricted or losing their elasticity due to atherosclerosis. In hypertensive retinopathy, fluids gradually seep out of weakened blood vessels into the spaces within the structure of the retina. This blood eventually clots and forms scar tissue, which pulls on the structure of the retina, causing blindness in extreme cases.

Standard treatment of hypertensive retinopathy is directed at resolving the basic problem (high blood pressure) and preventing progression of the disease. Preventing the development of hypertension should be the primary goal of all persons at risk for the disease—that is, those persons with the risk factors discussed above or a family history of the disease. The first step in treating hypertensive retinopathy is to recognize the presence of the disorder. Signs of this condition may show up early in the disease process, and prompt treatment may reduce the severity of eye complications.

NUTRITIONAL SUPPLEMENTS

Supplement	Directions for Use	Comments
Calcium and magnesium	1,500 to 3,000 mg of a combination supplement daily.	Deficiencies have been linked to hypertension.
Coenzyme Q_{10}	100 mg daily.	Improves heart function and lowers blood pressure.
L-carnitine, L-glutamic acid, and L-glutamine	500 mg of a combination supplement twice daily. Take on an empty stomach.	Aids in prevention of heart disease.
Lecithin	1,200 mg 3 times daily.	Emulsifies fat in the body and lowers blood pressure.
Selenium	100 mcg daily.	Deficiency has been linked to heart disease.
Vitamin C	3,000 to 6,000 mg daily.	Improves adrenal function and reduces blood clotting.
Vitamin E	200 IU daily.	Improves heart function.

HERBS AND HERBAL SUPPLEMENTS

Herb	Directions for Use	Comments
Cayenne	As directed on label.	Boosts circulation.
Fennel	As directed on label.	Anti-inflammatory.

Herb	Directions for Use	Comments
Garlic	250 mg 3 times daily.	Effective at lowering blood pressure.
Hawthorn	As directed on label.	Boosts circulation.
Hops	As directed on label.	Promotes relaxation the smooth muscles.
Lady's slipper	As directed on label.	Good for relaxation.
Parsley	As directed on label.	Relieves mucous discharge.
Passion flower	As directed on label.	Good for relaxation.
Rosemary	As directed on label.	Stimulates skin.
Scullcap	As directed on label.	Relieves smooth muscle spasm.
Valerian	As directed on label.	Calms nerves.

HOMEOPATHIC REMEDIES		
Remedy	Directions for Use	Comments
Crataegus oxycantha 6c	20 drops of tincture in 4 ounces of water. Use daily for three months.	Regulates blood pressure.
Lachesis 6c	3 to 4 pellets under the tongue 3 to 4 times daily.	Increases vascular integrity.
Natrum muriaticum 6c	3 to 4 pellets under the tongue 3 to 4 times daily.	Good for increased salt intake.

RECOMMENDATIONS

- Consider lifestyle counseling, a program to revamp your way of living. Lifestyle counseling will address your eating habits, exercise routine, stress level, work habits, and more.

- Have your blood pressure checked at least every four to six weeks. If necessary, buy your own blood pressure-checking equipment. Many pharmacies have self-test equipment available for public use.

- People with high blood pressure often have sleep apnea. If you have this condition, consult your physician.

- Nitric oxide is a powerful vasodilator, which lowers blood pressure.

The human body takes nitrates from vegetables and converts them into nitric oxide.

- Lose weight. Of all the natural methods of lowering blood pressure, losing weight is definitely the most effective. On average, a ten-pound loss of weight lowers blood pressure readings by as much as five points.

- Exercise more. Exercise helps by boosting weight loss but is also beneficial in its own right. The usual goal is at least thirty minutes of aerobic exercise three times a week. Weightlifting and bodybuilding are not recommended.

- Cut down on your alcohol intake. More than one or two drinks a day raise blood pressure.

- Reduce your salt intake because it lowers nitric oxide production.

- Increase your potassium intake. Fruits and vegetables are good sources of potassium and are also low in sodium.

- Try reducing stress levels.

- Quit smoking.

IRITIS

Iritis is an inflammation of the iris that sometimes includes the ciliary body. There are many causes of iritis, and even when the disorder is treated early, it can reoccur, unfortunately. In most cases, however, it eventually disappears completely.

Iritis is often related to a disease or infection in another part of the body. Diseases such as arthritis, tuberculosis, and syphilis may contribute to its development. Iritis may occur following an injury to the eye or if an ulcer or foreign body injures the cornea. Symptoms of iritis usually appear suddenly and develop rapidly over a few hours or days. Iritis commonly causes extreme pain, redness, tearing, light sensitivity, and blurred vision. Floaters can be another symptom.

Your doctor should do a careful eye examination when symptoms of iritis occur. Typically, a blood test, skin test, or X-ray should be done, and other specialists may be consulted to determine the cause of the inflammation. The most conventional treatment of iritis is the use of steroid drops and ointments to relieve the pain, quiet the inflammation, and reduce any scarring that may occur. Antibiotics may be prescribed. In severe cases, oral medications and injections may be necessary.

A case of iritis usually lasts about two months. During this time, patients must be observed carefully for side effects from the medications and any complications that may arise. Cataract, glaucoma, corneal changes, or secondary inflammation of the retina may occur as a result of iritis or its treatment.

Nutritional recommendations are listed to support the primary medical treatment of this condition.

NUTRITIONAL SUPPLEMENTS

Supplement	Directions for Use	Comments
Boron	3 mg daily.	Supports connective tissue.
Bromelain	As directed on label.	Assists in the production of prostaglandins.
Evening primrose oil	As directed on label.	Assist in the production of prostaglandins.
Fish oil	3,000 mg daily (EPA and DHA).	Anti-inflammatory.
Superoxide dismutase (SOD)	As directed on label.	Antioxidant.
Vitamin B$_5$	500 mg daily.	Assists in the production of steroid hormones.
Vitamin E	200 IU daily.	Antioxidant.

HERBS AND HERBAL SUPPLEMENTS

Herb	Directions for Use	Comments
Belladonna	As directed on label.	Dilates pupil.
Curcumin	375 mg 3 times a day.	Anti-inflammatory.
Cat's claw	As directed on label. (Do not use during pregnancy.)	Good for pain.
Feverfew and ginger	As directed on label. (Do not use feverfew during pregnancy.)	Good for pain and soreness.

HOMEOPATHIC REMEDIES		
Remedy	Directions for Use	Comments
Aconite 6c	3 to 4 pellets under the tongue 3 to 4 times daily.	Good for iritis in early stages.
Allium cepa 6c	3 to 4 pellets under the tongue 3 to 4 times daily.	Good for inflammation.
Apis mellifica 6c	3 to 4 pellets under the tongue 3 to 4 times daily.	Alleviates swelling.
Belladonna 6c	3 to 4 pellets under the tongue 3 to 4 times daily.	Good for inflammation accompanied by dilated pupils.
Calcarea fluorica 6c	3 to 4 pellets under the tongue 3 to 4 times daily.	Good for inflammation accompanied by light sensitivity.
Euphrasia officinalis 6c	3 to 4 pellets under the tongue 3 to 4 times daily.	Good for all eye conditions.
Mercurius corrosivus 6c	3 to 4 pellets under the tongue 3 to 4 times daily.	Alleviates pain and inflammation.
Rhus toxicodendron 6c	3 to 4 pellets under the tongue 3 to 4 times daily.	Good for inflammation accompanied by muscle paralysis.

RECOMMENDATIONS

• If you are diagnosed with iritis, keep your eyes "quiet"—that is, avoid light, wind, dust, sun, and other types of irritants.

MACULAR DEGENERATION

Age-related macular degeneration (AMD) is the main cause of blindness in older adults. It also responds to nutritional intervention very well. Released in 2001, the Age-Related Eye Disease Study (AREDS) used a combination of antioxidant supplements containing 500 mg of vitamin C, 400 IU of vitamin E, and 15 mg (or 25,000 IU) of beta-carotene, in addition to 80 mg of zinc and 2 mg of copper. Its results showed a 25 percent reduction in risk of advanced AMD. This treatment, however, was developed in the late 1980s, and emerging science has shown other nutritional ingredients to be effective in supporting retinal health.

Results of a follow-up study, AREDS2, were released in 2014. This study used the original AREDS formula as a placebo and added lutein, zeaxanthin, and omega-3 fatty acids to create a new therapy. While the research showed a positive effect from the lutein and zeaxanthin but not from the fish oil, these results were complicated and applied only to later-stage disease. It is a landmark study, however, and these substances should be considered in the treatment of AMD.

Of interest are the macular pigments lutein and zeaxanthin, which are lacking in the US diet. These carotenoids support skin, retinal, and crystalline lens health. They are found in abundance in the macula, where they sharpen vision, enhance contrast, and reduce glare. The antioxidant and filtering abilities of these substances may protect the outer retina from oxidative damage. Lutein, zeaxanthin, and vitamins E and C may work synergistically to inhibit lipid peroxidation, thereby allowing omega-3 fatty acids to exert their protective effects on photoreceptor cells in the retina.

Like all carotenoids, lutein and zeaxanthin are fat-soluble, and therefore require dietary fat for absorption and transport. Too much of the body fat known as adipose tissue, however, inhibits these actions, and the nutrients get stored in this tissue instead. Women and obese people require a higher intake of these carotenoids than do men or thinner individuals. A number of observational studies have indicated that dietary lutein and zeaxanthin may have a protective effect against AMD.

Lutein and zeaxanthin are found in egg yolk, and in leafy greens such as spinach, kale, and collards. They are moderately plentiful in vegetables such as bell peppers and broccoli. There is mounting evidence that increased consumption of lutein and zeaxanthin improves macular pigment optical density, indicating an important role in preserving vision and supporting retinal function.

Risk factors for AMD include age, diet and nutrition, sunlight exposure, smoking habits, heredity, and heart disease. In addition, women are more likely than men to suffer from AMD, and Caucasians more likely than African Americans.

NUTRITIONAL SUPPLEMENTS

Supplement	Directions for Use	Comments
Eye and Body Complete (Biosyntrx)	3 capsules twice a day.	Balanced formula.

Supplement	Directions for Use	Comments
Longevinex	As directed on label.	Supports retinal function.
Selenium	400 mcg daily.	Antioxidant.
Vitamin A	3,000 IU daily. (Use the emulsion form for easier assimilation and greater safety.)	Antioxidant.
Vitamin C with bioflavonoids	1,000 mg 4 times daily. (Use powdered buffered ascorbic acid.)	Antioxidant.
Vitamin E	200 IU daily.	Antioxidant.
Zinc	25 mg daily. (Do not take more than 40 mg daily. Use zinc monomethionine form.)	Deficiency has been linked to eye problems.

HERBS AND HERBAL SUPPLEMENTS

Herb	Directions for Use	Comments
Bilberry	160 mg daily.	Improves retinal function.
Blueberry	Drink 8 to 10 ounces of tea daily.	Rich in flavonoids.
Ginkgo biloba	As directed on label.	The dry form stimulates blood flow in capillaries.

HOMEOPATHIC REMEDIES

Remedy	Directions for Use	Comments
Hamamelis virginiana 6c	3 to 4 pellets under the tongue 3 to 4 times daily.	Alleviates venous congestion and vascular infiltration.
Lachesis 6c	3 to 4 pellets under the tongue 3 to 4 times daily.	Good for macular degeneration with muscle fatigue.
Phosphorus 6c	3 to 4 pellets under the tongue 3 to 4 times daily.	Good for many eye conditions. Improves tissue metabolism and reduces vascular and blood degeneration.

RECOMMENDATIONS

- While you can't stop the aging process, you can watch your diet. Eat a well-rounded diet with lots of fresh vegetables and fruit, and a minimum of processed foods.

- Increase your consumption of legumes, yellow vegetables, flavonoid-rich berries (such as blueberries, blackberries, and cherries), and foods rich in vitamins C and E (such as raw fruit and vegetables).

- Avoid alcohol, cigarette smoke, sugar, saturated fat, and food containing fat or oil that was subjected to heat or exposed to air, including fried food, hamburgers, luncheon meat, and roasted nuts.

MULTIPLE SCLEROSIS

Multiple sclerosis (MS) is an inflammatory disease of the body's central nervous system. This disease destroys the protective myelin sheath around nerves. It appears that MS is most likely some form of autoimmune disease, and may even originate with a viral infection. Multiple sclerosis can affect the optic nerve, causing vision problems that range from mild symptoms to changes in color vision, scotomas, or even complete blindness. It can also affect extraocular muscles, causing eye disorders such as diplopia from strabismus, poor binocular coordination, and possibly nystagmus. Very often, in fact, these visual problems are the first signs of MS.

MS is usually diagnosed between the ages of twenty-five and forty. Women are affected nearly twice as often as men. MS is rarely diagnosed in children or people over sixty years of age. There is no single diagnostic test for the disease, so diagnosis must be done by ruling out other possible causes of the symptoms.

Fortunately, most people with MS have periods of remission during which their symptoms improve or even disappear. Many years can go by before serious visual impairment occurs—and it may not occur at all. Systemic steroids and other medications are now used to improve symptoms of multiple sclerosis, including associated eye problems. There is no known cure for MS, but the following supplement and dietary recommendations have proven helpful in alleviating symptoms. Long-term sufferers of MS may not benefit as much, but younger people who are only starting to exhibit symptoms may find that the correct supplements slow or even stop progression of the disease.

NUTRITIONAL SUPPLEMENTS

Supplement	Directions for Use	Comments
Choline and inositol	As directed on label.	Stimulate central nervous system and protect myelin sheath.
Coenzyme Q_{10}	100 mg daily.	Boosts circulation and improves tissue oxygenation. Strengthens immune system.
Gamma-linolenic acid or BioTears (Biosyntrx)	As directed on label.	Essential fatty acids may help to control MS symptoms. Deficiency is common in MS.
Sulfur	500 mg 2 to 3 times daily.	Protects against toxic substances.
Vitamin B complex	100 mg 3 times daily.	Aids immune function and maintains healthy nerves.
Vitamin B_6	50 mg 3 times daily.	Promotes red blood cell production and supports nervous system and immune function.
Vitamin B_{12}	1,000 mcg twice daily. (Use sublingual form.)	Supports cellular longevity and prevents nerve damage by maintaining myelin sheath.
Vitamin D_3	5,000 IU daily.	Deficiency possibly related to MS development.

HERBS AND HERBAL SUPPLEMENTS

Herb	Directions for Use	Comments
Alfalfa	As directed on label.	Good source of vitamin K.
Burdock, dandelion, echinacea, goldenseal, red clover, St. John's wort, sarsaparilla, taheebo, and yarrow	As directed on label.	Excellent detoxifiers.
Garlic	1,000 mg 3 times daily.	Excellent source of sulphur.
Lobelia, skullcap, and valerian	As directed on label. (Take at bedtime.)	Calm nerves and prevent insomnia.

HOMEOPATHIC REMEDIES		
Remedy	Directions for Use	Comments
Aurum 6c	3 to 4 pellets under the tongue 3 to 4 times daily.	Good for pain.
Gelsemium sempervirens 6c	3 to 4 pellets under the tongue 3 to 4 times daily.	Good for headache with fever.
Hyoscyamus 6c	3 to 4 pellets under the tongue 3 to 4 times daily.	Relieves spasm.
Natrum muriaticum 6c	3 to 4 pellets under the tongue 3 to 4 times daily.	Good for pain.
Nitricum acidum 6c	3 to 4 pellets under the tongue 3 to 4 times daily.	Good for pain.

RECOMMENDATIONS

- Eat only organically grown foods that have not been chemically treated and contain no chemical additives, including eggs, fresh fruit, gluten-free grains, raw nuts and seeds, fresh vegetables, and cold-pressed vegetable oils. The best diet for people with multiple sclerosis is vegetarian.

- Eat foods that contain lactic acid, including sauerkraut and dill pickles. Substances with lots of chlorophyll are also beneficial, including dark green leafy vegetables.

- A strong immune system may ward off development of MS by assisting the body in avoiding infection, which often precedes onset of the disease.

- Once a diagnosis is confirmed, educate yourself and your family about the disease, and seek out sources of emotional support. Watch your diet, take your supplements, and try to maintain a positive attitude and a clean lifestyle.

MYOPIA

There is no cure for myopia, or nearsightedness. Myopia is the most common refractive error in humans, affecting over 32 percent of the population of the United States, and up to 80 percent in Asia. It most often starts in childhood and continues to worsen until early adulthood, at which time, absent other stress factors, it generally stabilizes. Heredity may be a factor in this condition, as studies have shown a tendency for myopia to develop more often in the children of myopic parents. Myopia is also much more prevalent in societies whose people do a lot of close work. In other words, the more reading and near-point work a society does, the higher its incidence of myopia tends to be.

In children, myopia increases along with the amount of time spent focused on near-point activities. Close to 2 percent of children entering school in the United States are myopic to some degree. That figure only increases with age. While it is generally believed that the progression of myopia stabilizes by a person's early twenties, doctors are now seeing myopic progression well into the late twenties and even thirties. Computers are almost certainly one of the culprits of this change. They require constant near-point focus, and more children and adults are spending more time in front of them.

Research has shown that blood levels of vitamin D from sunlight are 20 percent lower in myopic children than in non-myopic children. We know that vitamin D participates in cell signaling, works with retinoic acid (which changes the rate of eye growth), and potentially affects refractive error. This concept is still considered emerging science, but the potential looks positive.

There is probably no escape from activities that require near-point focus. During grade-school years, children read the equivalent of about 700 books. When this reading time is added to play time and computer time, it's not hard to see why so many people develop myopia. Surveys have shown that children between eight and eighteen years old spend over seven hours a day viewing digital images. It appears unlikely that this condition will be resolved any time soon.

NUTRITIONAL SUPPLEMENTS		
Supplement	Directions for Use	Comments
Calcium	800 mg daily. (Take with Vitamin D3.)	Important in collagen formation.
Chromium	80 to 100 mg daily.	Deficiencies have been found in persons with myopia.
Copper	1 mg daily.	Important in collagen formation.
Vitamin A	3,000 IU daily.	Good for all eye conditions.

Supplement	Directions for Use	Comments
Vitamin C	2,500 mg daily.	Strengthens collagen for stronger eyes.
Vitamin D$_3$	5,000 IU daily.	Affects cell signaling for eye growth.

RECOMMENDATIONS

- Once your children begin attending school, have their eyes checked regularly. Make sure near vision is tested.

- When doing near-point activities, take regular breaks to give your eyes a rest.

- Increase your intake of fiber and reduce your intake of simple carbohydrates. Avoid most processed foods.

- If you are sick with fever, try to avoid near-point activities. High temperatures weaken and soften collagen, which can easily become stretched with increased eye pressure.

NYCTALOPIA

True night blindness is a relatively rare condition in the United States. The main symptom of this disorder is a decrease in visual acuity under nighttime viewing conditions. Most often, night blindness is caused by a nutritional deficiency—specifically of vitamin A—and is common in underdeveloped countries. Vitamin A is necessary for the formation of rhodopsin, a light-sensitive receptor protein. Other causes of night blindness are fatigue, emotional disturbances, and hereditary factors.

It is also very common for individuals who are just beginning to become myopic to complain of difficulty seeing clearly at night. This is different than true night blindness. More likely they suffer from transient induced myopia and not true nyctalopia.

Zinc deficiencies are associated with diminished night vision, usually due to zinc's importance in vitamin A metabolism. Additionally, it competes with copper for absorption, so balancing these two minerals is imperative. Drugs that increase levels of inositol triphosphate have been shown to increase cellular debris in the eye. Taking inositol with vitamin D may be beneficial in the treatment of nyctalopia.

Eating bilberries is often mentioned as way to sharpen night vision. This belief was made popular by a story concerning British RAF pilots who had supposedly sharpened their vision by eating bilberries and, in doing so, had defeated the enemy. Although the effect of bilberry on night vision is unconfirmed, studies in rats have provided some evidence that bilberry consumption may inhibit or reverse eye disorders such as macular degeneration. Bilberries are certainly a good source of flavonoids, some of which have antioxidant activity. Nevertheless, they should not be considered an effective therapy for night vision problems at this time.

There are some very serious eye conditions whose main symptom is night blindness, most notably retinitis pigmentosa. Supplementation to support this symptom is dictated by the cause of the condition.

NUTRITIONAL SUPPLEMENTS

Supplement	Directions for Use	Comments
Copper	1 mg daily.	Must be used if zinc is taken.
Inositol	2,000 mg daily.	Combine with 1,000 mg vitamin D_3.
Vitamin A	3,000 IU daily.	Supports the retina.
Vitamin B complex	75 to 100 mg daily.	Good for nerve function.
Zeaxanthin	8 mg daily.	Improves contrast sensitivity.
Zinc	25 mg daily.	Good in combination with vitamin A.

RECOMMENDATIONS

- Have a complete eye examination once a year. Regular examinations can catch night blindness before it becomes disabling.

- In general, supplementing your diet with vitamin A will help to protect your eyes against night blindness. In addition, vitamins B_1, B_2, and B_3, as well as zinc may relieve night blindness if vitamin A does not produce a response.

OPTIC NEURITIS

Optic neuritis is an inflammation of the optic nerve. It can also manifest as retrobulbar neuritis. Optic neuritis is generally experienced as an acute blurring or loss of vision, almost always in one eye, although occasionally in both eyes. The visual deficit usually reaches its maximum within a few days and generally improves within eight to twelve weeks.

It has been estimated that about 55 percent of patients with multiple sclerosis have an episode of optic neuritis. Frequently, optic neuritis is the first symptom of MS. A study reported that persons with optic neuritis who also had abnormalities in their spinal fluid were more likely to develop MS. Other studies have demonstrated that a majority of patients with optic neuritis show signs of demyelination in the brain. While other disease processes can cause optic neuritis, in a young, otherwise healthy person, MS is the most likely cause.

Corticosteroids are the standard treatment for this condition. When a B complex or B_1 deficiency is responsible for optic neuritis, supplementing with these vitamins will result in recovery within three to four days. B vitamins must be taken in adequate amounts even when a deficiency doesn't exist, however, since they are needed for the general health of nerve tissue.

A well-balanced diet is necessary for effective repair and maintenance of muscles and nerves. Whenever you have an infection, you should boost your caloric, protein, and fluid intakes.

NUTRITIONAL SUPPLEMENTS

Supplement	Directions for Use	Comments
Fish oil	3,000 to 5,000 mg daily (EPA).	Anti-inflammatory.
Glutathione	500 to 1,000 mg daily.	Supports nerve and brain tissues.
Lecithin	2 tbsp twice daily. (Use granular form.)	Protects and repairs nerves.
Magnesium	400 mg daily.	Supports B complex vitamins.
Protein	1/3 g for every 1 pound of body weight daily.	Important for the repair of body tissue.
Vitamin B complex	At least 100 mg daily.	Good for nerve function.

HERBS AND HERBAL SUPPLEMENTS

Herb	Directions for Use	Comments
Bilberry	60 mg daily.	Antioxidant.

Herb	Directions for Use	Comments
Oats	As directed on label.	Calms nerves. Soothes mucous membranes.
Skullcap	As directed on label.	Calms nerves. Relieves spasm.
St. John's wort	As directed on label.	Anti-inflammatory. Repairs and rebuilds nerves.
Valerian	As directed on label.	Calms nerves. Relieves spasm.

HOMEOPATHIC REMEDIES

Remedy	Directions for Use	Comments
Aconite 6c	3 to 4 pellets under the tongue 3 to 4 times daily.	Good for optic neuritis in early stages. Good for pain and inflammation.
Apis mellifica 6c	3 to 4 pellets under the tongue 3 to 4 times daily.	Good for inflammation.
Hypericum perforatum 6c	3 to 4 pellets under the tongue 3 to 4 times daily.	Reduces nerve irritability.
Phosphorus 6c	3 to 4 pellets under the tongue 3 to 4 times daily.	Good for many eye conditions.
Spigelia 6c	3 to 4 pellets under the tongue 3 to 4 times daily.	Good for pain and nerve sensitivity.

RECOMMENDATIONS

- Relaxation is a key component of the healing process. Reduce stress levels in all areas of your life.

- Avoid stimulants such as coffee, soft drinks, and cigarettes.

- Increase your fluid intake.

- Eat fresh fruit and vegetables, as well as raw nuts and seeds.

PINGUECULA

A yellow or white deposit on the conjunctiva, a pinguecula is thought to be caused by exposure to excessive UV light, dust, or wind, and is common in outdoor workers, such as farmers, gardeners, lifeguards, surfers, and construction workers. As they do not affect vision, these deposits do not need to be immediately removed. Pingueculae tend to swell when irritated, but they return to a stable condition once the irritant has been removed. There is currently no medical treatment for pingueculae. The presence of a pinguecula indicates that the eye is under environmental stress, and that some action needs to be taken to remedy the situation. In general, conventional treatment for this condition is to reduce irritation to the eye. Many doctors recommend over-the-counter eye lubricants, but these are simply palliative in nature.

Pingueculae have abnormal tear coverage over their surfaces. Nutritional support is directed towards supporting the tear film and anterior ocular surface.

NUTRITIONAL SUPPLEMENTS		
Supplement	Directions for Use	Comments
BioTears (Biosyntrx)	As directed on label.	Maintains proper tear film.
Vitamin A	5,000 IU daily.	Supports epithelial cells.
Vitamin C	2,000 to 6,000 mg in divided doses daily.	Protects the eye and supports tissue healing.
Zinc	25 mg daily.	Enhances immune response.

HERBS AND HERBAL SUPPLEMENTS		
Herb	Directions for Use	Comments
Chamomile	Apply as a hot compress or use as an eyewash.	Soothes eye tissue.
Eyebright and fennel	Apply as a hot compress or use as an eyewash.	Good for inflammation.

HOMEOPATHIC REMEDIES		
Remedy	Directions for Use	Comments
Apis mellifica 6c	3 to 4 pellets under the tongue 3 to 4 times daily.	Relieves swelling around the eyes.
Pulsatilla 6c	3 to 4 pellets under the tongue 3 to 4 times daily.	Good for eyelids that are stuck together.

Remedy	Directions for Use	Comments
Ruta graveolens 6c	3 to 4 pellets under the tongue 3 to 4 times daily.	Good for red eyes.
Sulphur 6c	3 to 4 pellets under the tongue 3 to 4 times daily.	Good for red eyelids.

RECOMMENDATIONS

• Watch your cholesterol levels. Some experts feel that a pinguecula might indicate high cholesterol. No research, however, has been conducted to explore this connection.

• Be sure to wear sunglasses that block UV light at all times when in outdoor conditions.

• Soothing eyewash is the best remedy to quiet a pinguecula that has become irritated. Use the previously mentioned herbal remedies as eyewashes. Do not use eye drops intended to whiten the eye. Stay out of irritating environments and wear sunglasses when outdoors for extended periods of time. If your eyes feel dry, follow the suggestions in the section on dry eyes.

PTERYGIUM

A benign growth on the white of the eye, a pterygium is commonly mistaken for a pinguecula. It is also believed to grow in response to exposure to ultraviolet light. It is more common in light-skinned people living nearer the equator, particularly where outdoor activities are popular. As a pterygium grows, it replaces the corneal epithelium and erodes the superficial layers beneath it. The pterygium pulls and distorts the cornea as it enlarges. Pterygia are often associated with blepharitis.

No exact cause of this condition is known, but it occurs more frequently in hot, dusty climates, and it is often seen among surfers, who spend hours in the windy ocean spray and sun. Nutritional support is directed towards supporting the tear film, conjunctiva, and corneal surface.

NUTRITIONAL SUPPLEMENTS		
Supplement	Directions for Use	Comments
BioTears (Biosyntrx)	As directed on label.	Supports the tear film and anterior ocular surface.

Supplement	Directions for Use	Comments
Vitamin A	5,000 IU daily.	Good for epithelial cells.
Vitamin C	2,000 to 6,000 mg in divided doses daily.	Protects the eye and supports tissue healing.
Zinc	40 mg daily.	Enhances immune response.

HERBS AND HERBAL SUPPLEMENTS

Herb	Directions for Use	Comments
Chamomile	Apply as a hot compress or use as an eyewash.	Soothes eye tissue.
Eyebright and fennmel	Apply as a hot compress or use as an eyewash.	Boost circulation.

HOMEOPATHIC REMEDIES

Remedy	Directions for Use	Comments
Apis mellifica 6c	3 to 4 pellets under the tongue 3 to 4 times daily.	Relieves swelling around the eyes.
Bellis perrenis	3 to 4 pellets under the tongue 3 to 4 times daily.	Helps with healing and capillary weakness.
Lachesis	3 to 4 pellets under the tongue 3 to 4 times daily.	Reduces inflammation.
Ruta graveolens 6c	3 to 4 pellets under the tongue 3 to 4 times daily.	Good for hot, red eyes.
Sulphur 6c	3 to 4 pellets under the tongue 3 to 4 times daily.	Good for red eyelids

RECOMMENDATIONS

- Once a pterygium has started to grow, reducing your exposure to environmental irritants is the best thing you can do. Keep away from wind, dust, sun, and smoke. In addition, keep your eyes lubricated and moist.

- Wear good quality sunglasses that completely block UV radiation.

RECURRENT CORNEAL EROSION

Recurrent corneal erosion is a condition in which the epithelial cells of the cornea fail to adhere to their basement membrane following a corneal abrasion, resulting in pain, heightened sensitivity to light, the feeling of a foreign body in the eye, and tearing. The mildest approach to treating this disorder is to use artificial tears or a temporary antibiotic. This also might include the use of a lubricating ointment at bedtime to prevent the eyelids from sticking to the loose corneal cells. If this approach is not successful, a bandage contact lens may be used to protect the cornea from physical contact with the eyelids. If the scratch is deep, a pressure bandage may be required.

Nutritional supplementation is directed at supporting the corneal surface and the tear film. Hyaluronic acid plays an important role in the treatment process due to several of its properties.

NUTRITIONAL SUPPLEMENTS

Supplement	Directions for Use	Comments
BioTears (Biosyntrx)	As directed on label.	Supports anterior surface of the eye.
Hyaluronic acid	As needed. (Use eyedrop form.)	Aids epithelial cell integrity.
Vitamin A	3,000 IU daily.	Supports corneal tissue.
Vitamin C	500 mg 3 times daily.	Builds collagen tissue.

HERBS AND HERBAL SUPPLEMENTS

Herb	Directions for Use	Comments
Aloe vera liquid	Use as an eyewash daily.	Increases mucins.
Bayberry, eyebright, and goldenseal	Use as an eyewash twice daily. (Do not take goldenseal internally for more than 1 week. Do not use goldenseal during pregnancy.)	Good for all eye conditions.
Comfrey	Use as an eyewash.	Promotes healing.
White willow bark	400 mg as needed.	Good for pain.

HOMEOPATHIC REMEDIES		
Remedy	**Directions for Use**	**Comments**
Aconite 6c	3 to 4 pellets under the tongue every 3 to 4 hours, or put 2 drops in 1 cup of water and use as an eyewash.	Good for pain and inflammation.
Hypericum perforatum 6c	3 to 4 pellets under the tongue every 3 to 4 hours, or put 2 drops in 1 cup of water and use as an eyewash.	Reduces effects of nerve injury.

RECOMMENDATIONS

- Keep your eyes well lubricated at all times. Even during sleep, the lids may creep apart, allowing the eye to dry out to some degree. If necessary, use surgical tape to keep the lids closed while sleeping.

- Avoid sunny, windy, dusty, or other drying environments.

RETINITIS PIGMENTOSA

Retinitis pigmentosa (RP) is a term used to describe a cluster of inherited retinal diseases that can begin at any time from infancy through late middle age. RP is characterized by a progressive loss of rod and cone cells. Rods begin to die first, often in adolescence, causing night blindness. As this condition progresses, peripheral vision may be lost by young adulthood. Finally, central vision is lost later in life.

Although there is no cure for RP yet, there may be some means of slowing its progression. Research suggests vitamin A palmitate may slow the decline of retinal function in RP patients. Combining vitamin A and DHA supplementation may also be helpful. Some scientists also point to lutein as a protective element, stating that if a sufferer of retinitis pigmentosa were to add lutein to vitamin A and fish oil supplementation before the age of forty, peripheral visual field sensitivity would remain normal for an additional three to ten years. Some forms of RP are believed to be a result of chronic copper toxicity. Thus, copper-chelating drugs have been proposed as treatment. The addition of zinc to the diet can achieve a similar result.

Retinitis pigmentosa shares some features with AMD, including the degeneration of photoreceptor cells and the death of retinal pigment epithelial cells. Both diseases may also involve oxidative stress-mediated injury. It is therefore not surprising that a few of the nutrients thought to be protective in AMD may also be of value to RP patients.

NUTRITIONAL SUPPLEMENTS		
Supplement	Directions for Use	Comments
Fish oil	3,000 mg daily (at least 1,000 mg DHA).	Supports rod function.
Inositol	2,000 mg daily.	Combine with 1,000 mg vitamin D_3.
Lutein	20 mg daily.	Supports rod function.
Vitamin A	15,000 IU daily. (Use emulsion form for easier assimilation and greater safety.)	Good for all retinal conditions.
Zinc	25 mg daily.	Aids in the transport of vitamin A and supports immune system.

HOMEOPATHIC REMEDIES		
Remedy	Directions for Use	Comments
Nux vomica 6c	3 to 4 pellets under the tongue 3 to 4 times daily.	Good for nerve inflammation.
Phosphorus 6c	3 to 4 pellets under the tongue 3 to 4 times daily.	Supports nerve and vascular integrity.

RECOMMENDATIONS

- There is no treatment for retinitis pigmentosa offered by the medical community. Practitioners recommend getting in touch with a low-vision clinic and using the best low-vision aids you can obtain.

- Genetic counseling is also in order for any inherited disorder.

STYE

An external stye is an infection of sebaceous glands at the base of the eyelashes or of sweat glands found on the margins of the eyelid. Styes appear as small red bumps on the outside of the eyelid, though they may also form underneath the eyelid. They have an acute onset and most go away within a week or so, but a stubborn one may be incised and drained. Topical antibiotics may also be used.

There are some over-the-counter remedies for styes that contain mercuric oxide. These remedies may work, but the mercury in these preparations can be very irritating to the eye, causing itching, stinging, and redness. For this reason, use of these products is not recommended. Nutritional support is directed towards anti-inflammatory nutrients.

NUTRITIONAL SUPPLEMENTS

Supplement	Directions for Use	Comments
Fish oil	3,000 mg daily (EPA and DHA).	Anti-inflammatory.
Vitamin A	5,000 IU daily.	Good for all external eye conditions. Especially beneficial if styes are a frequent problem.

HERBS AND HERBAL SUPPLEMENTS

Herb	Directions for Use	Comments
Eyebright	Apply as a compress or use as an eyewash.	Good for all eye conditions.
Raspberry	Apply as a compress or use as an eyewash.	Alleviates redness and irritation.

HOMEOPATHIC REMEDIES

Remedy	Directions for Use	Comments
Apis mellifica 6c	3 to 4 pellets under the tongue 3 to 4 times daily.	Alleviates swelling.
Graphites 6c	3 to 4 pellets under the tongue 3 to 4 times daily.	Good for styes accompanied by severe discharge.

Remedy	Directions for Use	Comments
Lycopodium 6c	3 to 4 pellets under the tongue 3 to 4 times daily.	Good for styes accompanied by severe discharge.
Pulsatilla 6c	3 to 4 pellets under the tongue 3 to 4 times daily.	Good for styes accompanied by mucous discharge. Especially good for styes in upper eyelids of children. Good for inflammation.
Sepia 6c	3 to 4 pellets under the tongue 3 to 4 times daily.	Good for styes accompanied by watery discharge.
Staphysagria 6c	3 to 4 pellets under the tongue 3 to 4 times daily.	Good for lumps in eyelids. Especially good for recurrent styes. Supports connective tissue. Good for inflammation.
Sulphur 6c	3 to 4 pellets under the tongue 3 to 4 times daily.	Good for recurrent styes. Good for inflammation.

RECOMMENDATIONS

- Do not attempt to drain the head of a mature stye. Doing this can lead to more serious problems. Instead, contact your doctor for proper treatment.

- In early stages, use a hot compress several times a day.

SUBCONJUNCTIVAL HEMORRHAGE

The blood vessels that appear on the sclera, or white of the eye, are actually embedded in a membrane called the conjunctiva. If these blood vessels leak for any reason, blood will be released into the space between the membrane and the sclera. The blood will be very visible to the observer but will never spill out of the eye.

This condition is a benign disorder and a common cause of red eye. The major risk factor in young patients is trauma, while common causes in the elderly include systemic vascular diseases such as hypertension, diabetes, and arteriosclerosis. If the problem recurs or persists, further evaluation—including testing for systemic hypertension, bleeding disorder, or ocular malignancy—is warranted.

Nutritional therapy is directed towards supporting anterior eye tissue as well as blood vessel strength.

NUTRITIONAL SUPPLEMENTS

Supplement	Directions for Use	Comments
Calcium and magnesium	1,000 to 1,500 mg of a combination supplement daily.	Essential for blood clotting.
Vitamin A	5,000 IU daily.	Good for all anterior segment conditions.
Vitamin B complex	100 mg daily.	Lowers homocysteine levels.
Vitamin C	3,000 mg daily.	Important for blood clotting and strengthening blood vessel walls.
Vitamin K	120 mcg daily.	Helps with coagulation.

HERBS AND HERBAL SUPPLEMENTS

Herb	Directions for Use	Comments
Alfalfa	As directed on label.	Good source of vitamin K.
Spinach	1 cup daily.	Good source of vitamin K.

HOMEOPATHIC REMEDIES

Remedy	Directions for Use	Comments
Arnica montana 6c	3 to 4 pellets under the tongue 3 to 4 times daily.	Good for subconjunctival hemorrhage caused by injury. Reduces hemorrhaging and venous congestion.
Sanguinaria 6c	3 to 4 pellets under the tongue 3 to 4 times daily.	Improves vasomotor activity and reduces congestion.

RECOMMENDATIONS

- If you experience subconjunctival hemorrhages frequently, especially without apparent cause, you should consult your internist for a blood test.

- Apply a cold, wet washcloth as a compress to the affected eye when you first notice a subconjunctival hemorrhage. Repeat several times during the first twenty-four hours.

- No treatment other than a cold compresses on the first day is necessary during the first forty-eight hours.

- On the fourth day, begin applying a warm compress to the affected eye. A warm compress will hasten the breakdown of visible blood.

CONCLUSION

All healing requires nutritional balance in the body. We must remember that the eyes are an integral part of the body and will manifest problems if disease occurs. While many people feel they get an adequate amount of essential nutrients through diet, it is more likely that they are deficient in at least a few vitamins and minerals. In reality, for most individuals, a well-formulated nutritional supplement is likely appropriate—not as a substitute for good diet but rather as a safety net to ensure the necessary tools for proper healing are present.

PART THREE

Nutritional Approaches

Using a nutritional approach to support eye health is more than just popping a few pills. It is about a number of lifestyle changes that can help to heal not just the eyes but the entire body as well. These new habits to your daily routine include eating nutritious whole foods, getting sufficient exercise, and, when needed, taking dietary supplements. In addition to vitamin and mineral supplementation, herbal therapy may also prove useful, and homeopathy can offer a method you may not have considered. This section takes a closer look at the basics of diet and outlines many of the well-known diets out there. It also explores the effects of various nutritional supplements and sheds light on the concepts of herbal medication and homeopathy.

DIET

For most people, the word "diet" is synonymous with starvation, restriction, and a miserable lifestyle. The fact that nutritional advice is often confusing and frustrating only compounds this negativity. One day, a certain food or supplement is good for you; the next day, it is not. Nevertheless, the truth remains that the food you eat plays a major role in all aspects of your health.

The body requires energy to function. It gets its energy by taking in food, digesting it, and metabolizing its components. The food that you eat contains energy from the sun, which has been captured and stored by green plants and then passed along to fruits, seeds, and animals. Basically, you eat these foods and burn the fuel they contain.

These days, people have almost infinite food choices. You have no doubt heard, however, that there are "good" foods and "bad" foods, and that many authorities say we eat too much food. When you think of it, the concept of health food is actually a sad statement on what is available at the typical grocery store. Why would there even be such a section? Shouldn't all food be healthy?

So, is it the amount of food people eat or is it something else that has created the obesity epidemic we now face? There are many determinants of health, including genetics, environment, and social and spiritual factors. Diet is only one aspect of lifestyle, and lifestyle is only one aspect in the mix when it comes to health. Of course, while you are more than just what you eat, it would be beneficial to take a look at some of the more common diets to see how you can use food to help, not hurt, your waistline and your health.

Proper nutrition for good vision and eye health in particular means eating a diet that activates health-promoting genes and deactivates disease-promoting genes. You cannot change your genes, but you can control the expression of the genes behind some chronic diseases. You can do this by choosing the foods that support health rather than those that create illness. Unfortunately, the typical American diet—high in processed items, junk food, refined grains, sugar, salt, and chemical additives—tends to turn on genes that promote inflammation and chronic disease. When dietary habits affect genes that control the eye, they can result in conditions such as macular degeneration, cataract, dry eye, or hypertensive retinopathy.

Diet Basics

Due to genetic differences from person to person, there may not be one ideal diet for everyone, but there are some general dietary concepts that have proven to be beneficial overall. For example, despite the misconception that eating fat makes you fat, fat is required by the body. Moderate amounts of fat from wild animals and fish, nuts, and seeds provide a good source of energy and the right balance of building materials for healthy cells and nerves. Saturated fat and grain-based polyunsaturated omega-6 fat, however, contribute to inflammation.

Complex carbohydrates, of course, are needed for their fiber and to maintain stable levels of blood glucose and insulin in the body. But the modern diet is overloaded with unhealthy refined grains, starches, and sugars. These foods are digested and absorbed rapidly, causing blood sugar and insulin levels to rise quickly. These rapid elevations in sugar and insulin result in quick declines in sugar and insulin in the blood, which lead to unstable blood sugar levels, and possibly to disease processes such as diabetes. Complex carbohydrates, which are metabolized much more slowly than simple sugars, are preferred, as they do not cause such drastic spikes in blood sugar levels.

Cereal grains contain natural chemical substances called phytates, which can inhibit absorption of vitamins and minerals. Unless grains are properly prepared by soaking, sprouting, or fermenting them to neutralize phytates and other toxins, they can contribute to nutrient deficiencies. Many native people used soaking and fermenting techniques as food preservation methods, benefiting from the enhanced bioavailability of proteins, vitamins, and minerals that resulted from these practices. A good example of this idea is associated with soy. While raw soy products can be problematic due to their estrogenic effects, fermented soy (tempeh, miso, etc.) can be a powerful source of protein and other healthful nutrients. Food made from refined cereal grains today has been fortified with minerals and synthetic vitamins, in part to offset the antinutrient effect of phytates and similar substances.

Basically, a moderate amount of healthful protein should be eaten with complex carbohydrates from fresh fruit and vegetables, as well as a reasonable amount of recommended fats. It's important to note that drinking fruit juice is not the same as eating a piece of fruit. The juice contains all the fruit sugar and none of the fiber needed to process the sugar appropriately.

A well-balanced diet should provide an abundance of essential vitamins, minerals, and phytochemicals such as carotenoids, bioflavonoids, and polyphenols, whose antioxidant and anti-inflammatory properties are vital for good vision and eye health.

Diet Programs

There are over sixty studies linking excessive weight to chronic eye disease. Diet is clearly linked to eye health, but the number of diet plans out there makes it seem impossible to find the best one for your body. Your eyecare practitioner or nutritionist can guide you in choosing the right food plan, which will benefit not only your eyes but your life in general.

Atkins Diet

The Atkins diet, which has been around since the 1960s, has gained worldwide attention as a way to eat a lot of food, not be hungry, and still lose weight. Atkins relies on the theory that carbohydrates cause weight gain by eventually turning into fat, and that it is possible to eat a lot of protein and fat while your weight decreases by simply eliminating or strictly limiting carbohydrates. Without carbohydrates, the body is forced to convert fat into energy, which is an inefficient process. The body uses its fat stores at a faster rate, resulting in weight loss. This theory seems beneficial to dieters who have trouble metabolizing carbohydrates.

The Atkins diet, however, has received its fair share of criticism, and for good reason. It recommends eating greater amounts of animal protein and fat, and these foods cause water to be lost from the body, placing strain on the kidneys, which are usually weakened in diabetics. The Atkins diet is also thought to increase the chance of heart disease due to its high red meat content. Finally, the Atkins diet can lead to dangerously low blood sugar levels (hypoglycemia). For a person with diabetes, extremely low blood sugar can lead to a coma. Most experts agree that using the Atkins diet for diabetes can be risky and should not be attempted without medical permission and supervision.

While a traditional approach to weight loss focuses on limiting refined sugar and foods that convert into sugar, this type of diet may contain an unhealthful amount of fat and protein.

Ketogenic Diet

Ketogenic diets are very high in fat and very low in carbohydrate and protein. This concept is similar to the Adkin's diet (in fact, some of the latest research shows that a modified Atkins diet is just as good as the keto-genic diet). The classic ketogenic diet uses a ratio of 4:1:1 for fat, carbo-hydrate, and protein. Some people consider ketogenic diets to be extremely difficult and unappetizing, whereas low-carb dieters tend to find such discouragement silly.

Speaking of fat, you may be confused about fat and its possible neg-ative impacts on health. Controversy regarding this subject exists even among healthcare professionals. The fact is that all forms of fat are not cre-ated equal. The key word here is "created," as some saturated fats occur naturally, while others are artificially created, such as the saturated fat that comes from the process of hydrogenation. Hydrogenation manipu-lates vegetable and seed oils by adding hydrogen atoms while heating these substances. This act produces thickened oil that benefits the shelf life of processed foods and gives these edibles a firmer texture. The medical and scientific communities are now fairly united in the opinion that hydrogenated vegetable and seed oils should be avoided. The artificial fats created by hydrogenation are called trans fats. There is no controver-sy regarding the health dangers of these artificial compounds any longer. While the FDA continues to take steps towards eliminating trans fats in food products, you should make the right choices to avoid them as well.

Mediterranean Diet

Based on food patterns typical of Crete, much of the rest of Greece, and southern Italy in the early 1960s, the Mediterranean diet emphasizes abundant amounts of plants, fresh fruit, olive oil, and dairy products (principally cheese and yogurt). It also encourages moderate intake of fish, poultry, and eggs, and a low intake of red meat. Red wine is also con-sumed in reasonable amounts. Total fat in this diet makes up approxi-mately 30 percent of calories, with saturated fat accounting for about 8 percent of this amount.

Studies have shown that type 2 diabetics on a Mediterranean diet may be better able to manage the disease without medication than those who eat a low-fat diet. One study on diabetics compared the Mediterranean diet with a low-fat diet and found that only 44 percent of the Mediter-ranean-diet subjects needed their medications, as opposed to 70 percent of the followers of a low-fat diet.

There is an inverse association between adherence to the Mediter-ranean diet and the incidence of fatal and nonfatal heart disease in initially healthy middle-aged adults in the Mediterranean region. While dietary factors are a part of the reason behind the health benefits of the Mediterranean diet, a healthy, physically active lifestyle also plays a large role.

Paleo Diet

The Paleolithic diet, or Paleo diet, is based on the premise that modern humans are genetically suited to the diet of their Paleolithic ancestors, and that human genetics have barely changed since the dawn of agriculture. Therefore, the ideal diet for human health and well-being, it is said, is one that resembles this ancestral diet. For almost all of human evolutionary history, humans and human ancestors survived on hunter-gatherer diets.

Proponents of this diet argue that modern humans eating diets similar to those of Paleolithic hunter-gatherers are largely free of what they consider the diseases of affluence, such as diabetes. Supporters point to several nutritional characteristics of this type of diet, including its reliance on lean meat, seafood, vegetables, fruit, and nuts, and its low content of cereals and dairy products. It is also high in unsaturated fatty acids, dietary cholesterol, and several vitamins. Studies have concluded that a Paleolithic diet may improve glycemic control and several cardiovascular risk factors as compared to the typical diabetic diet. Because they ate wild game, including organ meats and brains, our Paleolithic ancestors consumed higher amounts of omega-3 fatty acids and lower amounts of omega-6 fatty acids. They also had higher vitamin D levels as a result of the sun exposure they received from spending more time outside. These substances can have powerful effects on health.

Raw Food Diet

An extension of the vegan diet, the raw food diet consists of unprocessed, raw plant foods that have not been heated above 40 °C (104 °F). Raw foodists believe that food cooked above this temperature has lost much of its nutritional value and is less healthful (perhaps even harmful) to the body. The argument is: Raw or living food has natural enzymes, vitamins, and minerals, which are necessary to build proteins and maintain good health within the body, and the process of heating food kills these beneficial substances and may even leave toxins behind. Typical items included in the raw food diet are fruit, vegetables, nuts, seeds, and sprouted grains and legumes.

Raw foodists believe that items such as coffee, alcohol, and tobacco are irritants and poor choices in regard to this type of diet. In addition, heated fat and protein, including fried oil and roasted nuts are to be avoided, as they are considered carcinogenic.

As is the case with most extreme diets, the raw food diet can be challenging to maintain. There is no question that raw food has qualities that make it desirable in any quest to become healthy, but ever since man discovered fire, much of our food has been cooked, and this process has provided benefits as well. As always, balance in diet is the best option.

Vegetarian Diet

The reduced level of fat in the vegetarian diet helps insulin to be more effective in the body. Research has found that patients on oral medications or insulin were able to discontinue use of these substances after twenty-six days on a near-vegetarian diet and exercise program. In addition, soy-based food, which often plays a major role in the vegetarian diet, can lower cholesterol, decrease blood glucose levels, and improve glucose tolerance in people with diabetes. Found in soy, bioactive compounds called isoflavones may exert antidiabetic effects by targeting fat cell-specific factors and downstream-signaling molecules important in the process of glucose uptake.

Vegetarianism offers numerous other health benefits. It is heart-healthy. Because there is no animal fat, there is almost no cholesterol. (While I maintain that some cholesterol in the diet is not only harmless but actually desirable, some people produce excessive cholesterol internally and need to exert some control in this area.) Moreover, a vegan diet, which does not include dairy, eliminates casein, the dairy protein found in milk. Casein is a common trigger for rheumatoid arthritis and joint pain. Another advantage of vegetarianism and veganism is that the food eaten in these diets contains high levels of fiber and nutrients, which help people to lose weight and lower blood pressure.

Nutrition for Diabetics

Diabetes mellitus, commonly referred to as diabetes, is diagnosed when a group of metabolic conditions result in elevated blood sugar levels over a prolonged period of time. High blood sugar can lead to many health problems, including cardiovascular disease, kidney disease, foot ulcers, and eye troubles. While type 1 diabetes, which most often occurs in young people, has no known cause, type 2 diabetes, which typically arises during adulthood, has been linked to weight problems and lack of exercise primarily.

Due to its connection to eye problems, diabetes is a significant issue for eyecare providers to consider. Millions of Americans have diabetes, and millions have been diagnosed with a collection of conditions considered "pre-diabetes." This condition costs the US healthcare system hundreds of billions of dollars every year. Cases of adult-onset, or type 2, diabetes are more prevalent in people between the ages of forty and sixty, although diagnosis of type 2 has been growing at an alarming rate in people under the age of eighteen. Diabetes is the seventh leading cause of death and the leading cause of blindness in adults. Diabetic retinopathy causes thousands of cases of blindness each year and is associated with increased cardiovascular events.

The diabetes epidemic has been fueled by increasing rates of overweight and obesity, leading to the term "diabesity." While eyecare providers may focus time and energy on how to treat the ocular complications associated with diabetes, it is important to learn how to prevent type 2 diabetes before these issues arise. Education on nutrition is of paramount importance. There are many ideas regarding what the proper diet might be for a type 2 diabetic who is overweight. Depending on this condition's severity and length of existence, varying amounts of protein, fat, fiber, and carbohydrate are recommended. Consult your physician or nutritionist for advice on nutrition if you are considering changing your dietary habits.

Coconut Oil

The body uses medium-chain fatty acids as an additional source of energy. This makes coconut oil (the most common source of medium-chain fatty acids) a powerful means of instant energy—a function usually served in the diet by simple carbohydrates. Although coconut oil and simple carbohydrates can both deliver quick energy to the body, only coconut oil does not produce an insulin spike. It acts like a carbohydrate, but without any of the insulin-related effects associated with long-term high-carbohydrate consumption. Diabetics and prediabetics should immediately realize the benefit of coconut oil. In fact, coconut oil added to the diets of these patients may actually help to stabilize weight gain, likely decreasing the likelihood of these patients getting type 2 diabetes.

Coconut oil also increases the activity of the thyroid, enhancing the metabolic rate. It is commonly known that a sluggish thyroid is one reason why some people are unable to lose weight, regardless of which diet they follow. Other advantages to boosting the metabolic rate include accelerated healing and an immune system that functions better overall. Because much of the saturated fat contained in coconut oil is in the form of lauric acid, coconut oil is a better alternative to partially hydrogenated vegetable oil when solid fat is required.

Supplements

Supplementation is expected to benefit people with diabetes. It is surprising that major diabetes organizations make no supplement recommendations except in cases of known deficiency. Still, there is accumulating evidence that supplementation with certain vitamins, minerals, essential fatty acids, antioxidants, and botanicals might ward off complications of diabetes. For those diabetics considering supplements to treat eye problems, few guidelines are ever suggested, as eyecare providers may not be comfortable doing so. Nevertheless, these substances have proven helpful:

- **Alpha-lipoic acid.** Alpha-lipoic acid is a "super antioxidant" that preferentially distributes to mitochondria. It blocks glycosylation of protein, improves glucose transport to insulin-dependent tissues, and reduces both small and large blood vessel complications of diabetes in animal models.

- **Benfotiamine.** Benfotiamine is a synthetic derivative of vitamin B_1 that is mainly sold as an antioxidant. It reduces activity in all four biochemical pathways implicated in microvascular complications of diabetes.

- **Carotenoids.** Patients who demonstrate high levels of circulating carotenoids in blood plasma are much less likely to develop diabetic retinopathy than those with low levels.

- **Chromium.** Chromium is an essential mineral that may improve insulin sensitivity and lower blood sugar levels in type 2 diabetics.

- **Coenzyme Q_{10}.** CoQ_{10} may help to improve blood sugar levels. It may also aid in the management of high blood pressure in diabetics.

- **Curcumin.** Curcumin is the compound that gives the spice turmeric its yellow coloring. It has been shown to reduce insulin resistance and improve the status of insulin-producing cells in the pancreas.

- **Omega-3 essential fatty acids.** Omega-3 fatty acid supplements have been shown to prevent cardiac arrhythmias, improve clinical depression in type 2 diabetic patients, and reduce peripheral insulin resistance.

- **Pycnogenol.** This standardized extract of French maritime pine bark contains substances that appear to lower blood sugar, improve blood vessel function, and fight inflammation.

- **Resveratrol.** This natural substance found in certain plants may improve glucose control and insulin sensitivity in diabetics. It may also reduce oxidative stress.

- **Taurine.** This amino acid supports retinal health. High doses may lower blood glucose levels.

- **Vitamin D.** Vitamin D deficiency impairs insulin sensitivity and has been associated with type 1 and 2 diabetes.

- **White mulberry.** White mulberry is a small mulberry tree that has white or pinkish fruit. The leaf of white mulberry may benefit diabetics, as its extract may inhibit high blood sugar levels and the formation of arterial plaque.

Exercise

Scientists have long known that those who change their lifestyles by eating healthier, losing weight, and exercising more, also lower their chances of developing type 2 diabetes. In 2002, the National Institute of Diabetes & Digestive & Kidney Diseases (NIDDK), which forms part of the National Institutes of Health, confirmed this point of view when it released the findings of the Diabetes Prevention Program (DPP). This multicenter clinical research study aimed to determine if lifestyle modification or treatment with an oral diabetes drug, metformin, could prevent or delay the onset of type 2 diabetes. Its results were quite positive. According to the NIDDK, a high-risk person may avoid developing type 2 diabetes by losing 7 percent of his body weight and maintaining that loss by eating less fat and fewer calories, and by exercising for at least 150 minutes a week. In fact, the study found that diet and exercise interventions reduced the risk of a person developing type 2 diabetes by 58 percent. Lifestyle changes were shown to be particularly effective in people sixty years old and up. The study also found that metformin helped forestall onset of the disease, reducing risk by 31 percent. This effect was mostly seen in young people with weight problems.

Researchers have studied the long-term effects of intensive lifestyle interventions on the incidence of type 2 diabetes in those with impaired glucose tolerance. Over the course of six years, twenty minutes a day of moderate exercise coupled with a diet rich in vegetables and low in alcohol and sugar delayed the onset of type 2 diabetes in at-risk subjects for as long as fourteen years. Preventing diabetes is about lifestyle changes— mainly smart dietary habits and regular physical activity. Too many individuals do not take diabetes as seriously as they should. On average, this condition shortens life by almost ten years, and significantly reduces quality of life. Individuals with high-fat diets who consume far more calories per day than they need and don't exercise at all seem not to understand that such a lifestyle is literally killing them.

In addition to lifting weights and doing cardiovascular workouts, other examples of ways to increase daily physical activity level include taking the stairs instead of an elevator or escalator, walking instead of driving whenever possible, parking farther away from a destination, and

Glycemic Index

The glycemic index (GI) ranks carbohydrate levels in foods on a scale from 0 to 100 according to the extent to which they raise blood sugar levels. Items with a high-GI (over 55), such as fruit juice, contain carbohydrates that are rapidly digested and absorbed, resulting in a spike in blood sugar and an excess of insulin in the bloodstream. Low-GI foods (under 55), which have carbohydrates that produce a more gradual rise in blood sugar and insulin levels, allow the body to use up the glucose from the breakdown of these foods before it gets stored in fat cells as glycogen. When excess fat is stored, it enlarges fat cells in adipose tissue and increases the risk of chronic diseases such as diabetes and cancer. As a result, low-GI foods have proven benefits for health.

While the GI is an important concept, the glycemic load (GL) may, in fact, be more so. The GL measures a food's effect on blood sugar by taking into account how much carbohydrate exists in a particular portion size of that food, giving the user a more accurate idea of the extent to which that food will raise blood glucose. For example, while the GI of watermelon is high (i.e., its carbohydrates are rapidly absorbed), the actual carbohydrate content of watermelon is relatively low, which gives the fruit a low GL. Essentially, a small quantity of a food with a high glycemic index will have the same effect on blood sugar as a large quantity of a food with a low glycemic index. The lower a food's glycemic load, the better.

taking a walk every few hours as a break from remaining sedentary for so long.

HERBAL THERAPY

Herbs are plants that lack the woody characteristics of shrubs and trees. Over the years, many important compounds have been extracted from a variety of herbs, as well as from other types of plants, and used successfully to heal the human body. Herbs can be therapeutic food for the body. They contain vitamins and minerals, and often possess medicinal properties. They have a remarkable history of curative effects when used properly. Herbs have been used for centuries, and many of today's modern medicines, in fact, have their foundations in herbal therapy, or herbalism.

The exact reasons for the positive effects that herbs exert on the human body are not always known. It is evident, however, that the nutrients stored within plants' cellular structures are in forms that are easily metabolized by the body. The therapeutic actions of herbs come from alkaloids, which are organic compounds that cause certain chemical reactions within the body. Alkaloids also help the body to resist disease, strengthen tissue, and improve the nervous system. It is an often-overlooked fact that the organic chemical structures of hemoglobin (the substance within red blood cells that carries oxygen and gives blood its red color) and chlorophyll (the substance within green plants that absorbs light and gives plants their green color) are very similar in molecular structure.

In this discussion of herbs and herbal therapy, you will find the most popular herbs used as eye therapy, as well as the most common Western herbal combinations and traditional Chinese herbal combinations used to treat eye problems.

Western Herbs Vs Chinese Herbs

Herbs are grown all over the world but some of the more popular are Chinese herbs. In China, unlike in other parts of the world, herbalists have sought out special tonic herbs that can be taken daily to improve physical condition, enhance energy, increase resistance to disease, and prolong life. These herbs in particular help to distinguish Chinese herbalism from other forms of the art, such as Western herbalism. The term "Western" as used in herbalism really applies to methods of using herbs rather than to origins of herbs. This is why Western herbalism books often list substances from places such as Asia, Africa, South America, and Egypt. Individual herbs are used for their reputed health benefits, not because of the way they may act against a complex health syndrome or interact with other herbs in a combination formula.

Chinese herbalism, also known as Traditional Chinese Medicine (TCM), arranges physical signs and symptoms into patterns of organ disharmony, which can then be treated with acupuncture and herbal combinations to restore harmony and balance in the human body. The treatment of disease by TCM is generally a complicated procedure and should be performed by an experienced practitioner. The herbal formulas are often adjusted as the symptoms change during recovery. Some of these formulas are meant for short-term therapy only. There are several patented medicines made in China and the United States that can be used to treat vision problems and benefit overall health. A healthcare professional trained in TCM should oversee their usage.

Forms of Herbal Preparations

Herbal preparations can be applied in many different forms. The best are the tincture and the extract, which remain potent longer than any other form. A tincture is an herb mixed in an alcohol solution. It is made by adding a powdered herb to alcohol and then adding enough water to make a 50-percent alcohol solution. After letting the mixture stand for two weeks, shaking the bottle once or twice a day, it may then be used after it has been strained. Herbal extract is procured by hydraulically pressing the herb and then soaking the pressed herb in alcohol or water. The excess liquid is allowed to evaporate and the result is a concentrated liquid. Before using an extract, dilute it in a small amount of water. Never use an alcohol-based extract, no matter how diluted it is, directly in the eye. A tincture should also not be used in the eye.

Capsules are a pleasant way to take herbs, especially when the herbs taste bitter or are mucous-forming. Capsules are generally made of gelatin and filled with the powdered herb. If prepared capsules are purchased from a first-class herb company or health food store, generally the herbs are clean and combined in the correct proportions. To comfortably wash down and properly dissolve a capsule, take it with eight ounces of pure water or herbal tea.

An herbal compress will achieve an effect similar to that of an oint-ment, but has the advantage of the therapeutic action of heat. To make a compress, bring one or two heaping tablespoons of the herb to a boil in one cup of water. Dip a cotton pad or piece of gauze in the strained liq-uid, let the excess liquid drain off, and place the pad or gauze over the closed eyelid while still warm. Keep the compress in place until it has cooled off.

An infusion is made by pouring hot water over dry or powdered herb and steeping the herb for several minutes, thus extracting its active ingre-dients. This method of preparation minimizes the loss of the herb's volatile elements. The usual amounts are about half an ounce to one ounce of herb to one pint of water. Use an enamel, stainless steel, porcelain, or glass pot with a tight-fitting lid to prevent evaporation and loss of the essential oils (the main medicinal part of some herbs). Steep the herb for about ten to twenty minutes. To drink an infusion, strain it into a cup and drink it lukewarm or cool. A decoction is similar to an infusion. Instead of steeping the dry herb, however, you would simmer it for about twen-ty to thirty minutes. Always be careful not to boil the herb.

Having herbal tea as a late-afternoon pick-me-up or just before bed to help release the tensions of the day has become as common in the United States today as tea time has been in England for centuries. But herbal tea can be used as more than a drink. Used as eyewash, an herbal tea infu-sion or decoction can bring relief to a stressed eye through the direct application of the properties that make the herb so beneficial.

To prepare an herbal tea or other mixture for external application to the eye, use a piece of cheesecloth or filter paper to strain the mixture repeatedly until it runs clear. In addition to being free of any debris that could scratch or irritate the eye, the mixture must also be allowed to cool to room temperature before being used. Any leftover liquid can be kept in the refrigerator for future use. Never use a mixture that is more than two weeks old.

A poultice is a warm, mashed, moist mass of fresh or ground herb tied in a piece of muslin or other loosely woven cloth. It is applied directly to the skin to relieve inflammation, boils, or abscesses, and to promote prop-er cleansing and healing of the affected area. Oil the skin before applying a poultice. Because the skin around the eyes is very thin, make sure the poultice is not too hot. A warm poultice is fine, but one that is too hot can easily cause a burn. Once a poultice has cooled, discard it. A cooled poul-tice should never be reheated and reused.

Best Herbs for the Eyes

There are nineteen herbs that are commonly used to treat eye conditions. In the following list, they are presented according to their most popular common names, with their Latin names following. Also included is general information on each herb, what the herbs contain nutritionally, what conditions they are used to treat, and how they affect the eyes.

Most herbs can be purchased in bulk from local health food stores or by mail order. When buying an herb, make sure that you have selected the correct variety, since quite a few herbs are known by more than one name. If you are unsure of the specific herb to buy, or of the action of an herb, consult an herbalist. It is best to store bulk herbs in airtight containers in a dark, cool place.

Alfalfa

Alfalfa (*Medicago sativa*) has been used for hundreds of years to treat kidney stones, and to relieve fluid retention and swelling. It is a perennial herb that grows throughout the world in a variety of climates. Alfalfa helps the body to assimilate iron, phosphorus, potassium, protein, calcium, and other nutrients. It contains high levels of chlorophyll, and is therefore a good body cleanser, infection fighter, and natural deodorizer.

The leaves of this plant contain eight essential amino acids. It is a good laxative and a natural diuretic. It is useful in the treatment of urinary tract infections, as well as kidney, bladder, and prostate disorders. Alfalfa alkalizes and detoxifies the liver. It promotes pituitary gland function and contains an antifungal agent. Finally, alfalfa is very rich in vitamins A, D, and K.

Bayberry

Bayberry (*Myrica cerifera*) can be useful in fighting off early signs of a cold, especially when taken along with the herb capsicum (*Capsicum frutescens*). It is also helpful when used as a gargle for tonsillitis and sore throat. It plays a role in the rejuvenation of the adrenal glands, cleansing of the bloodstream, and ridding of toxins from the system.

Bayberry has long been employed to restore the body to a healthy state and raise vitality and resistance to disease. It may also be used to aid digestion. Bayberry contains a high amount of vitamin C. It kills germs and is stimulating to the mucous membranes, especially those around the eye.

Bilberry

Bilberry (*Vaccinium myrtillus*) acts as a potent antioxidant, improves blood circulation (as a blood thinner), has anti-inflammatory properties, and enhances the regeneration of rhodopsin in the retina. It has been shown to be completely nontoxic, with no side effects and no contraindications (except in excess as a blood thinner).

The Bilberry plant is a small shrubby perennial that grows in the woods and meadows of northern Europe. Its berries have been used for centuries to make jams and jellies, but it wasn't until after World War II that its therapeutic benefits became known. Bilberry's fruit contains flavonoids and anthocyanin, which serve to prevent capillary fragility, thin the blood, and stimulate the release of vasodilators. Anthocyanin is a type of antioxidant that lowers blood pressure, reduces clotting, and improves blood supply to the nervous system. Bilberry also contains glucoquinine, which has the ability to lower blood sugar and is therefore helpful to diabetics.

Bilberry has long been promoted as a remedy for night blindness. This ability has not been confirmed. Some studies have shown it has a positive effect on night vision but others have not. Other promoted uses for bilberry include cataract, nearsightedness, diabetic retinopathy, eyestrain, macular degeneration, and glaucoma. While that description sounds miraculous, there is no one potion that heals everything, so use this tonic cautiously.

Borage Oil

Borage (*Borago officinalis*) is especially soothing in cases of bronchitis and digestive upset. It promotes activity of the kidneys and adrenal glands. It is soothing to the mucous membranes, including the conjunctiva. Borage tea can be used as an eyewash to ease ocular discomfort.

Borage oil contains gamma-linolenic acid (GLA), a fatty acid that the body converts into prostaglandin E1 (PGE1). PGE1 has anti-inflammatory properties and may also act as a blood thinner and blood vessel dilator. Linoleic acid, a common fatty acid found in nuts, seeds, and most vegetable oils, should theoretically convert to PGE1. Many things can interfere with this conversion, however, including disease, the aging process, saturated fat, hydrogenated oil, blood sugar problems, and inadequate levels of vitamin C, magnesium, zinc, or B vitamins. Supplements that provide GLA circumvent these conversion problems, leading to more predictable formation of PGE1. Borage also contains calcium and potassium.

Comfrey

Comfrey (*Symphytum officinale*) is one of the most valuable herbs known to botanical medicine. It has been used successfully for centuries as a wound healer and bone knitter. It feeds the pituitary with a natural hormone and helps to strengthen bones. It helps to maintain the calcium-phosphorus balance, which is important for strong bones and healthy skin. It encourages the secretion of the digestive enzyme pepsin, and is a general aid in digestion. It has a beneficial effect on all parts of the body and is therefore used as an overall tonic. Topically, comfrey was also used to treat minor skin irritation and inflammation. It has also been used as a wash or topical application for eye irritation and for treating conjunctivitis.

Comfrey is rich in vitamins A and C. It is high in protein, calcium, phosphorus, and potassium. It contains copper, iron, magnesium, sulfur, and zinc, as well as eighteen amino acids. Although comfrey root tea has been used traditionally, the danger of its pyrrolizidine alkaloids is significant. Therefore, comfrey root and young leaf preparations should not be taken internally.

Eyebright

Eyebright (*Euphrasia officinalis*), as its name suggests, has been used by herbalists primarily as a poultice for the topical treatment of eye inflammation, including conjunctivitis, blepharitis, and stye. Traditionally, a compress made from a decoction of eyebright is used to give relief from redness and swelling due to eye infections. A tea is sometimes given internally along with this topical treatment, but no studies have been conducted to confirm any internal effects. It has also been used for the treatment of eyestrain and other visual disturbances of vision. In addition, herbalists have recommended eyebright for problems of the respiratory tract, including sinus infection, cough, and sore throat.

While there are many chemicals that may be active in eyebright, no studies have shown any effect on eye inflammation or irritation. Some herbal texts suggest that the astringent actions of eyebright may reduce eye irritation while others suggest that eyebright may also have antibacterial effects topically. To date, there are no clinical studies to support or refute these proposed actions.

Eyebright is extremely rich in vitamins A and C. It contains the vitamin-B complex, vitamin D, and some vitamin E. It also has copper, iron, silicon, zinc, and a trace of iodine.

Ginkgo

Medicinal use of Ginkgo (*Ginkgo biloba*) can be traced back almost 5,000 years in Chinese herbal medicine. The nuts of the ginkgo tree were often recommended and used to treat ailments of the respiratory tract. The use of the leaves is a more recent development, originating in Europe.

In addition to supporting the cardiovascular system, ginkgo's antioxidant action may extend to the brain and retina. Some studies have suggested potential benefit for people with macular degeneration and diabetic retinopathy. Ginkgo may regulate the tone and elasticity of blood vessels, making circulation more efficient. It has been associated with increased circulation in the brain and other parts of the body, and may exert a protective action on nerve cells. If you have moderate or advanced AMD, however, ginkgo is contraindicated due to the potential for blood-vessel leakage associated with its use.

Ginkgo is most well known for its effect on memory and thinking. It may enhance cognition in healthy older adults, people with age-related cognitive decline, and people with Alzheimer's disease.

Goldenseal

Goldenseal (*Hydrastis canadensis*) has been used to boost a sluggish glandular system and promote youthful hormonal harmony. The active ingredient of the herb goes directly into the bloodstream and helps to regulate liver function. Goldenseal has a natural antibiotic ability to stop infection and kill poisons in the body. It is now considered an endangered species, and so is used rarely by responsible herbalists. It is also very expensive.

Goldenseal is valuable against all mucous-forming conditions in the nasal, bronchial, throat, intestinal, stomach, and bladder areas. It has the ability to heal mucous membranes anywhere in the body, including the external eye tissue. When taken with other herbs, its tonic properties are increased for whatever ailment is being treated.

Goldenseal contains vitamins A and C. It also has the B complex vitamins, vitamin E, calcium, copper, iron, manganese, phosphorus, potassium, sodium, zinc, and unsaturated fatty acids. There may be some negative interactions when taken with doxycycline or tetracycline antibiotics.

Hawthorn

Hawthorn (*Crataegus oxyacantha*) is a vasodilator that opens the blood vessels of the heart and also lowers cholesterol levels. In addition, it increases intracellular vitamin C levels and is useful against anemia, cardiovascular and circulatory disorders, high cholesterol, and lowered immunity. Hawthorn contains vitamins B_1, B_2, B_3, B_6, B_{12}, and C, as well as citric acid, choline, flavonoids, folic acid, PABA, and selenium. Hawthorn should not be taken with prescription drug Digoxin.

Marigold

Marigold (*Calendula officinalis*) is very useful as a first-aid remedy. It has been used as a tea for acute ailments, especially fever, and is effective as a tincture when applied to bruises, sprains, muscle spasms, and ulcers. It relieves earache, boosts heart function and circulation, and cleanses the lymphatic system. Traditionally, a sterile tea was topically applied in cases of conjunctivitis. It was discovered that the petals of the marigold flower have a significant amount of lutein, which is an important retinal pigment.

Marigold is high in phosphorus, and contains vitamins A and C. Flavonoids, found in high amounts in calendula, are thought to account for much of its anti-inflammatory activity. Other potentially important constituents include the triterpene saponins and carotenoids. The saponins are sugars that can be easily cleaved off in the gut by bacteria, allowing them into the cell membrane, where they can modify the composition, influence membrane fluidity and potentially affect signaling by many ligands and cofactors.

Passionflower

Passionflower (*Passiflora incarnata*) is used to treat insomnia and hysteria, as well as hyperactivity and convulsions in children. It is an herb that is quieting and soothing to the nervous system, and should be recommended to patients who wish to wean themselves from synthetic sleeping pills or tranquilizers. Passionflower helps to reduce high blood pressure and tachycardia, and is an effective antispasmotic. It is good for inflamed eyes. Passionflower contains bioflavonoids, and so exhibits anti-allergic, anti-inflammatory, antimicrobial, anticancer, and antidiarrheal properties.

Red Clover

Red clover (*Trifolium pratense*) is useful as a tonic for nerves and as a sedative for nervous exhaustion. Native Americans used the plant for sore eyes and as a salve for burns. It is useful mixed with honey and water as a cough syrup. It is also good as an aid in strengthening the immune systems of delicate children. Red clover is effective against cough, a weak chest, wheezing, bronchitis, lack of vitality, and nervous energy. It has also been included in some well-known cancer mixtures.

Red clover is a good source of vitamin A. It is high in iron, and contains the B complex vitamins, vitamin C, bioflavonoids, and unsaturated fatty acids. It is valued for its high mineral content. For example, it is rich in calcium, copper, and magnesium, and contains some cobalt, manganese, nickel, selenium, sodium, and tin.

Rose Hips

Rose hips (*Rosa canina*) are the fruit that develops after the pedals have fallen off the rose. They play an important role in treatments in which vitamins A, C, and E are needed. They are very nourishing to the skin. Rose hips contain a natural fruit sugar. They help to prevent infection, and also help when an infection has already developed.

Rose hips are very high in the vitamin-B complex, and are very rich in vitamins A, C, and E. (It is the herb with the highest vitamin C content.) They also contain vitamin D and bioflavonoids. Rose hips are high in calcium and iron. They also contain fair amounts of potassium, silica, sodium, and sulfur.

Rosemary

Rosemary (*Rosmarinus officinalis*) is a stimulant, especially of the circulatory system and pelvic region. It is considered a proven heart tonic, and is a treatment for high blood pressure. Rosemary is used externally on bites and stings. In cases of cold or flu, a warm infusion may be used early on. It may also be used as a cooling tea when symptoms include restlessness, nervousness, or insomnia. It has been considered one of the most powerful remedies to strengthen the nervous system. Rosemary is a good tonic for reproductive organs. It has also proven effective against diarrhea, especially in children.

Rosemary contains vitamins A and C. It is high in calcium, and also contains iron, magnesium, phosphorus, potassium, sodium, and zinc.

Rue

Rue (*Ruta graveolens*) has the ability to expel poisons from the system, and therefore has been used for snake, scorpion, spider, and jellyfish bites. It helps to remove deposits that tend to form in tendons and joints, especially wrist joints, with age. It has also been found to be effective in the treatment of high blood pressure and helps to harden bones and teeth.

Rue contains a large amount of rutin. Rutin is a bioflavonoid known for its ability to strengthen capillaries, arteries, and veins. It is also commonly used in its homeopathic form.

Sarsaparilla

Sarsaparilla (*Smilax officinalis*) is a valuable herb used to balance glandular function. Its stimulating properties are noted for increasing the metabolic rate. Sarsaparilla also contains precursors of both male and female hormones. It has been used to relieve sore eyes.

Sarsaparilla contains vitamins A, C, and D, as well as the B complex. It also has copper, iodine, iron, manganese, silicon, sodium, sulfur, and zinc.

Siberian Ginseng

Siberian ginseng (*Eleutherococcus*) is very effective at increasing circulation (especially around the heart), normalizing blood pressure, and combating stress and fatigue. It increases both brain efficiency and physical efficiency, and improves concentration span. It also strengthens adrenal and reproductive glands. Siberian ginseng contains the B complex, vitamin E, and eleutherosides, a type of complex sugar molecule with beneficial effects. It also stimulates T-cell production (supports the immune system) and improves lipid levels in the blood. It is a powerful antioxidant.

Taheebo

Taheebo (*Tabebuia*) also goes by the names pau d'arco, lapacho, and ipe roxo. It is found in South America, and is a very powerful antibiotic with virus-killing properties. Taheebo is said to contain compounds that seem to attack the causes of diseases. One of its main actions purportedly is to put the body into a defensive posture, to give it the energy needed for defense against and resistance to disease.

Taheebo contains a high amount of iron, which aids in the proper assimilation of nutrients and elimination of waste. In consideration of this fact, caution should be the rule when using this herb.

Wild Cherry

Wild cherry (*Prunus serotina*) is considered a very useful expectorant. It is a valuable remedy for all mucous-forming conditions and is beneficial against bronchial disorders caused by hardened accumulations of mucous. Wild cherry contains a volatile oil that acts as a local stimulant in the alimentary canal and aids in digestion. It is a useful tonic for persons convalescing from various chronic diseases. Wild cherry bark may be beneficial against the oxidative damage caused by free radicals due to its antioxidant properties.

Herbs to Avoid

Although you may reap positive effects from herbal remedies, you must still exercise caution as you use them. For example, the following herbs have the same anti-inflammatory effect as steroids—and can cause the same ocular problems, including cataract, glaucoma, herpes simplex keratitis, photophobia, and retinal blood vessel problems: beth root, damiana, fenugreek, ginseng, licorice, saw palmetto, blue cohosh, false unicorn root, figwort, goldenrod, red sage, and wild yam.

There are also some herbs that have the same beneficial effects as aspirin (salicylic acid), as well as the same harmful effects, including blurred vision, disturbed accommodation, optic atrophy, retinal edema, and visual field constriction. These herbs are birch, sweet violet, chickweed, black willow, pansy, meadowsweet, black cohosh, wintergreen, crampbark, and blue flag.

Diuretics affect the body's fluid and electrolyte balances. They can cause blurred vision, disturbed accommodation, dry eye, photophobia, xanthopsia, and myopia. Herbs that act as diuretics include bearberry, buchu, birch, bugleweed, blue flag, carline thistle, boldo, cleavers, broom tops, corn silk, shepherd's purse, parsley, stone root, pellitory-of the-wall, sweet violet, saw palmetto, wild carrot, sea holly, yarrow, couch grass, juniper, dandelion, licorice, fumitory, night blooming cereus, gravel root, pansy, and hydrangea.

Some herbs contain volatile or aromatic oils that can cause ocular effects including excessive tearing, irritation, contamination of contact lenses, and disorders of the central nervous system. These herbs are cinnamon, fennel, peppermint, rosemary, tansy, wild carrot, clove, garlic, prickly ash, self-heal, thuja, willow, cudweed, ginger, queen's delight, skunk cabbage, thyme, wintergreen, Echinacea, pennyroyal, red sage, southernwood, and valerian.

Some herbs have a drying effect on eye tissue. This can, in some cases, be detrimental, especially if you have dry eye or wear contact lenses. Some of these drying herbs are bistort, cudweed, eyebright, golden seed, mouse ear, pokeroot, coltsfoot, daisy, golden root, ground ivy, myrrh, and Scots pine.

Other herbs and their possible injurious side effects include:

- **Arnica:** eye irritation.

- **Bittersweet:** blurred vision, dilated pupils, loss of accommodation, glaucoma, and light sensitivity.

- **Bladderwrack:** metabolic changes due to altered thyroid activity.

- **California poppy:** constricted pupils.

- **Canthaxanthine:** abnormalities in visual field, retinal function, and dark adaptation.

- **Chamomile:** conjunctivitis.

- **Datura:** dilated pupils.

- **Echinacea:** eye irritation and conjunctivitis.

- **Ephedra:** dilated pupils, dry eyes, and increased eye pressure.

- **Gingo biloba:** retinal hemorrhage.

- **Kava:** blurred vision, redness, and dilated pupils.

- **Licorice:** transient visual loss.

- **Shepherd's purse:** blurred vision, red eyes, and constricted pupils.

- **Squill, figwort, hawthorn, lily of the valley, night-blooming cereus:** lazy eye, blurred vision, central blind spot, double vision, disturbed color vision, disturbed accommodation, and photophobia.

Herbs are naturally occurring substances in nature that have medicinal-type effects on the body. We can use herbs to treat disease, avoiding many of the negative side effects of pharmaceutical medication. But like medications, herbs can also be harmful if taken inappropriately. Therefore, you should take care when choosing an herbal therapy. I strongly recommend consulting a qualified herbalist before taking any herb.

Herbal Combinations

Herbal combinations have more than one function in the fight against eye problems. They consist of several substances that work together in natural harmony, each with its own benefit. When taken over a period of time, an herbal combination should condition the body to react in a way that is comparable to the manner in which it reacts to certain medications, albeit in a less drastic manner, and often without unwanted side effects. This is because herbs trigger neurochemical reflexes in the body that, over time, become automatic and continue even after the person stops using herbal therapy. One advantage of using an herbal combination instead of a medication is that herbs help the body to bring about its own recovery, making it unlikely to be susceptible to the same complaint during or after convalescence. Unlike pharmaceuticals, which treat symptoms, herbal combinations go right to the source of the disorder and treat its cause.

In regard to eye problems, two herbal combinations that work especially well are:

- **Bayberry, eyebright, and goldenseal.** Bayberry is high in vitamin C, kills germs, and stimulates mucous membranes. Eyebright boosts the body's immunity to eye problems. Goldenseal acts as a natural antibiotic against eye infection.

- **Bayberry, eyebright, goldenseal, raspberry, and capsicum.** In addition to the benefits of the first three substances, this combination has raspberry, which is effective against styes, acting as an astringent and helping to stop discharge. Capsicum acts as a stimulant and a relaxant. It is high in vitamin A and a number of minerals.

Bayberry, eyebright, and goldenseal are three of the more common herbs used for external eye conditions. Although each one used separately is effective, the combination benefits several types of eye conditions, making this combination a good choice if you are unclear regarding the condition from which you are suffering. Specifically, this combination may be supportive for cataract, iritis, conjunctivitis, and night blindness.

Use caution with the second combination listed. Capsicum is a very powerful herb and can cause severe damage to delicate tissue if not used properly. If the eye is very inflamed and has discharge, use a very small amount of capsicum in the mixture. This combination will help to increase circulation in the eye area and rid the tissue of toxins. Consult an herbalist if you have any concerns or questions about the proper combination of herbs to use.

When using an herbal combination, follow the same precautions for single herbs outlined earlier. A number of premixed herbal combinations are available from health food stores and by mail, but you may also mix a combination yourself if you are careful to keep your ingredients, tools, and work area clean. The typical recipe calls for approximately equal amounts of each herb. To prepare a tea, infusion, or other desired mixture, follow the procedures for single herbs already described.

Traditional Chinese Herbal Combinations for Eye Problems

Both a science and an art form, Chinese medicine is well over five thousand years old. Methods and procedures in Chinese medicine differ significantly from those in Western medicine. For example, a Chinese medical practitioner will generally ask different types of questions and perform different diagnostic tests than you might encounter in Western medicine. The emotional aspects of illness are often of more concern to Chinese practitioners than to Western practitioners, and the health interests of Chinese and Western practitioners frequently differ. Oftentimes, there is no correlation between Western medical terminology and that of traditional Chinese medicine.

Some traditional Chinese herbal combinations contain herbs chosen because of the way they interact with one another. It is rare for Chinese practitioners to use one herb alone. Some combinations include as many as twenty-five different herbs. A number of combinations also include non-herbal ingredients such as minerals, plants, or animal organs. Therefore, many of the combinations in the following list are not used strictly for eye conditions. Since Chinese medicine strives to treat the whole person—the body, mind, and spirit—treatment oftentimes is directed towards a whole other set of symptoms, which may or may not be apparent.

The Chinese use their observations of nature to describe the workings of the inner body. For example, a practitioner might talk about "heat from the liver" to describe a series of conditions caused by an emotional constraint or blockage of energy in the liver. This "heat from the liver" may manifest as an inflammation (a Western medical term) in the head area—for example, a sore throat or earache. A person's condition is a very individualized expression of a disorder, and different people may display completely different combinations of symptoms. The different combinations of symptoms that are possible are what have given rise to the various herbal combinations used in traditional Chinese medicine.

Since herbal preparations are not pure substances, you need to use caution when taking them. The problem is that different parts of the herbs—roots, leaves, pods, bark, seeds, and flowers—are often used, giving different batches varying degrees of potency. In some cases, the potency of the active ingredient in an herb exceeds that of the manufactured medication that uses the same ingredient. Furthermore, some companies package and market their products in a way that fosters misuse of natural products by consumers who believe that natural equals safe. The following list contains some of the more common traditional Chinese herbal combinations that may have beneficial effects on eye conditions.

EFFECTS OF CHINESE HERBS	
Chinese Herb	**Effects**
An mian pian	Cools liver "heat." Helps to relieve anxiety, red eye, and eye irritation.
Er ming zuo ci wan	Used to treat liver deficiency that is causing symptoms that include headache, high blood pressure, eye pressure, insomnia, thirst, and eye irritation.
Long dan xie gan wan	Used to purge liver and gallbladder "heat." Treats headache, red eye, and ringing in ears.
Ming mu di huang wan	Replenishes energy in the liver and kidneys. Used to treat dry eye, red eye, poor eyesight, light sensitivity, excessive tearing, and eye diseases such as glaucoma and cataract.
Ming mu shang qing pian	Dispels "heat," clears vision, and sedates the liver. Treats red eye, itching, tearing, and swelling.
Nei zhang ming yan wan	Benefits clarity of vision, nourishes the liver and kidneys, reduces "heat," and helps circulation. Use it to aid in recovery from eye surgery and for cataract, glaucoma, or itchy, painful eyes.
Niu huang shang qing wan	For systemic "heat" of the liver that causes headache, eye pain, red eye, sore throat, toothache, or fever.
Qi ju di huang wan	Nourishes kidneys. Improves blurred vision, dry eye, pressure behind eyes, and disturbed night vision. It may also be used to treat dizziness, headache, and restlessness.
Shi hu ye guang wan	Improves vision, especially eyesight that is beginning to become blurry. It is valuable in early stages of cataract formation. It is also suitable to treat tearing eyes, red eye, dry eye, and hypertensive changes within the eye.
Xiao yao wan	Treats stagnation of the liver due to a blood deficiency. Improves digestive dysfunction, menstrual and premenstrual disorders, vertigo, headache, fatigue, blurred vision, and red eye. It is also useful against allergies and hay fever.
Zhong guo shou wu zhi	An excellent tonic for the blood. It nourishes the liver and kidneys, and benefits eyes and tendons.

Of course, some products have undesirable side effects, which can lead to dire consequences. I highly recommend consultation with an experienced herbalist before taking any herb or herbal combination.

HOMEOPATHY

Homeopathic medicines are prescribed according to an age-old principle that recognizes the body's ability to heal itself. This is not a new approach to healing. This approach was formalized into a specific treatment modality in the early 1800s by a German physician named Samuel Hahnemann, but the system is older than even Hippocrates. It was extremely popular in the United States in the nineteenth century, and then declined because of new "wonder" drugs and political and economic changes in the practice of medicine. The holistic movement that surfaced in the early 1970s advocated a return to the natural laws of healing and sparked a revival of interest in this scientific system of medicine. Currently homeopathic medicine is regulated by the FDA as either prescription or over-the-counter drugs. The Homeopathic Pharmacopoeia of the United States (HPUS) dictates specifically how each medicine is sourced and manufactured. The FDA references the *Homeopathic Material Medica* to mandate which indications are allowed for each remedy.

Most medical practitioners brush off homeopathy as unscientific, or say that it produces nothing but a placebo effect. Many homeopaths, however, are medically trained and have seen the positive effects homeopathy can have on patients. What many Western doctors don't realize is that the remedies used in homeopathy don't actually heal the body but rather stimulate the body to heal itself. Essentially, it is a different way of looking at healing.

According to a report from the government of Norway, homeopathy is the most frequently used complementary and alternative medicine therapy in five out of fourteen European countries, including France, Belgium, the Netherlands, Norway, and Switzerland. In fact, homeopathic remedies are used by between 20 and 25 percent of Europeans. Homeopathy is so popular in Europe that it is no longer appropriate to consider it alternative medicine there.

In homeopathy, deciding which remedy to use for a specific condition starts with the patient's case history. Questions asked of the patient aren't as straightforward as you might think. For example, a homeopathic doctor might ask, "Is your skin dry, moist, hot, cool, sensitive, or clammy?" or, "Are you feeling anxious, frightened, stupefied, or confused?" These are not expected lines of investigation in Western medicine, but they actually allow a homeopathic physician to select the correct remedy. Western medicine's logic and protocol are not the only factors taken into account when a homeopath diagnoses physical disorders.

As with any science, the system of homeopathy is governed by certain laws that dictate how the process works. These laws must be followed in order for the process to be considered homeopathic. These laws are called the "Law of Similars," "Law of Proving," "Law of Potentization," and "Hering's Law."

The Law of Similars

The term "homeopathy" comes from the Greek words "homoios," meaning "similar," and "pathos," meaning "suffering" or "sickness." The concept of homeopathy is based on a foundation known as the Law of Similars, which states that "like is cured by like." According to this law, a treatment may cure a disease if that treatment produces symptoms similar to those of the patient's illness. This entire idea is attributable to Hindu sages from the tenth century BC, who poetically described this law as, "Through the like, disease is produced, and through the application of the like, it is cured."

A prime example of the Law of Similars is as follows: A person develops a fever accompanied by a flushed face, dilated pupils, a rapid heartbeat, and a feeling of restlessness. A homeopathic physician studies all these symptoms and then searches for a remedy that, under scientifically controlled conditions, has produced all these symptoms in a healthy person. After taking the remedy for a time, the patient's fever decreases and a feeling of wellness returns. In other words, using the Law of Similars, a doctor selects the medicine required by the patient by matching symptoms of the patient's disorder to symptoms the remedy is known to induce.

The Law of Proving

The second law of homeopathy, the Law of Proving, refers to the method used to test a substance to determine its medicinal effect. To prove a remedy, a dose of the test substance is given to half of a group of healthy people. The remaining people receive a placebo. Conforming to the standard double-blind method used in pharmacological experiments, neither subjects nor researchers know which substance a particular person has been given.

Every day, subjects carefully record any symptoms they may experience. When the proving is complete, it is determined who took what, and all symptoms experienced by the persons taking the substance are listed as a characteristic remedy picture in the reference book. To treat a patient, a physician looks up the remedy picture in the reference book and, when the symptoms fit, applies the Law of Similars.

The Law of Potentization

The Law of Potentization refers to the method of preparation of a homeopathic remedy. All homeopathic remedies are prepared using a controlled process consisting of dilution followed by succussion (shaking and striking on an elastic surface), which may be repeated until the resulting medicine contains few or no molecules of the original substance. These dilutions are called potencies. Lesser dilutions are known as low potencies, while greater dilutions are known as high potencies. Low potencies are used for more external conditions and acute conditions requiring repetition of dosage. Higher potencies are for chronic internal conditions as well as mental or emotional ones. As strange as it may seem, the more a remedy is diluted, the deeper acting is its potency. This is where most Western trained practitioners fail to see how homeopathy works. In traditional Western medicine, the more of the active ingredient in a solution, the more potent it is. In homeopathy, it is the opposite.

Potency is designated by a number followed by an "x" or "c." The "x" represents 10 and signifies that the original tincture has been diluted to 1 part in 10. The "c" represents 100 and signifies that the original tincture has been diluted to 1 part in 100. The original tincture is an alcohol-based extract of the substance, as it comes directly from the plant, animal, or mineral. The number preceding the "x" or "c" indicates the number of times the remedy has been diluted. Thus, a 3x-potency remedy has been diluted three times, and a 6x-potency remedy has been diluted six times. Tinctures and subsequent potencies are manufactured according to strict guidelines outlined by the Homeopathic Pharmacopoeia of the United States (HPUS). For purposes of consistency, the recommended homeopathic remedies in this book are all 6x and should be used three to four times daily.

When the process of potentization was devised roughly 200 years ago, the idea that medicine containing an infinitesimal amount of matter could be curative was inconceivable. In this nuclear and nanotechnological age, however, the power of minute quantities has been well established. The dose of vitamin B_{12} used to treat certain types of anemia contains one-millionth of a gram of cobalt. Trace elements, required for physical development and proper bodily function, are present in the body in barely measurable amounts. The human body manufactures between fifty-millionths and one-hundred-millionths of a gram of thyroid hormone each day, yet a small deviation in the amount produced can seriously affect the health of an individual.

The power of an infinitesimal dose is not clearly understood, but neither are the actions of many modern medications. The process of potentization makes it possible to use as medicines substances such as charcoal and sand, which are inert in their natural states. Potentized remedies do not contain sufficient matter to act directly on tissue, which means that homeopathic medicines are nontoxic and cannot cause side effects.

Hering's Law

Put forth by American homeopath Constantine Hering in the mid-nineteenth century, this law states that healing occurs in distinct patterns or directions: from above to below, from inside out, from the most to the least important organ, and in reverse order of when symptoms appeared.

A team of researchers at the University of Southampton in England conducted a study as a part of a larger investigation of homeopathic treatment of rheumatoid arthritis. They developed the "Hering's Law Assessment Tool" (HELAT)—a standardized way to gauge symptom progress during the course of homeopathic treatment. Their work found that the more a patient's symptoms followed the patterns of Hering's Law, the more that patient showed strong improvements in health and symptoms. Every single respondent had a high HELAT score, whereas the majority of the non-respondents had low HELAT scores. Nevertheless, a large number of nonrespondents had high HELAT scores. This seems to confirm that Hering's Law is more of a tendency than an ironclad phenomenon.

Combination Remedies

While homeopaths traditionally recommended only one remedy at a time, combination remedies have come into common usage. In fact, combination remedies have been utilized for several decades and have proven to be very effective. It is understood that if the incorrect remedy is given, nothing happens (no symptom similarity between the remedy and patient). A combination remedy works because one or more ingredients are similar to the patient's symptoms, causing self-regulating mechanisms in the body to respond in kind, while the other ingredients are not acknowledged by the immune system. By combining several ingredients into one remedy, the treatment has a higher chance of helping a broader range of condition variations, as well as a wider range of patients experiencing those symptoms.

Today, many homeopathic remedies are sold in health food stores under a description of symptoms—for example, "Cold," "Flu," or "Teething." Listed according to indications, the following combination remedies may prove as effective as single remedies.

HOMEOPATHIC REMEDY BY SYMPTOM	
Symptom	Remedy
Aching all over the body.	Gelsemium sempervirens
Any kind of shooting pain.	Hypericum perforatum
Blurred vision.	Lac caninum
Burning and irritation.	Euphrasia officinalis
Burning.	Arsenicum album; Magnesia carbonica
Cataract.	Cineraria maritima
Dilated pupils, light sensitivity.	Belladonna; Cinchona officinalis; Stramonium
Dimmed vision.	Agaricus
Discharge from any kind of infection.	Calcarea sulfurica
Double vision.	Aurum; Hyoscyamus; Magnesia phosphoric
Dry eye.	Arsenicum album; Veratrum album
Dryness associated with irritants, corneal erosion, or corneal abrasion.	Calendula officinalis

Symptom	Remedy
Dull vision.	Lachesis
Excessive tearing.	Sepia
Eye discharge.	Mercurius corrosivus
Eye infection.	Staphysagria
Eye injury, black eye, any kind of eye bruising.	Arnica montana
Eye pain accompanied by light sensitivity.	Silicea
Eye pain and tearing.	Lycopodium
Eye pain.	Aconite; Ledum palustre; Natrum muriaticum; Sanguinaria; Spigelia
Eyestrain followed by headache, red eye.	Ruta graveolens
Flickering lights.	Calcarea fluorica
Floater.	Cocculuc
Foggy vision.	Arsenicum album; Zincum metallicum
Gritty feeling in eyes.	Kali muriaticum
Headache (mostly in the forehead area).	Allium cepa
Headache.	Bryonia
Heavy eyes.	Conium
Inflammation of eye.	Antimonium crudum; Arsenicum album; Ferrum phosphoricum; Petroleum
Injury to the eyeball, pain from a blow to the eye.	Symphytum
Irritated eyes.	Cineraria maritima
Light sensitivity.	Graphites; Natrum sulfuricum; Nux vomica; Rhus toxicodendron
Muscle twitching.	Rheum
Muscle weakness.	Senecio
Pain.	Aurum

Symptom	Remedy
Red eye without discharge.	Mercurius vivus
Red eye.	Apis mellifica; Arsenicum album Belladonna; Ferrum phosphoricum; Glonoinum; Kali sulfuricum
Red eyelids.	Sulphur
Severe allergy.	Apis mellifica
Severe headache from stress.	Ignatia amara
Sticky eyelids with infection.	Argentum nitricum
Sticky eyelids with yellowish discharge.	Pulsatilla
Swelling around eyes.	Anacardium; Apis mellifica; Carboneum sulfuratum
Tearing.	Nitricum acidum
Tense eye muscles.	Cyclamen; Physostigma
Tired eyes.	Gelsemium sempervirens; Magnesia phosphorica
Tissue in need of calming.	Chamomilla
Tissue in need of purification.	Causticum

As shown, there may be many different remedies for the same symptoms. That is why a series of questions must be answered to determine which specific remedy is most appropriate for your condition. This type of approach takes extensive training and should only be used by a homeopathic physician or specialist.

Homeopathy Vs Herbal Therapy

Many people are confused about the differences between homeopathy and herbal therapy, as both systems use herbs as medicine. Herbalism uses herbs as natural pharmaceuticals or nutrients, homeopathy uses them to modulate the immune system and gently trigger the body's self-regulating mechanisms to respond in a healing manner. An herbalist may use an age-old formula for making an herbal tea or poultice, but, like a chef, may also improvise, personalizing the recipe. In addition, using intuition and experience, herbalists often combine a number of herbs to increase the effect desired. Homeopathy is somewhat more scientific, its remedies prepared, tested, and prescribed according to specific laws and procedures.

Some herbs by themselves are toxic, particularly when ingested in large amounts. Herbalists cannot use these herbs. Although many homeopathic treatments are made from poisonous herbs or plants, the potentized remedies contain only minute amounts of the original substances and are nontoxic. It cannot be overemphasized that caution should be taken with any remedy of any kind, of course. Although a homeopathic remedy may be harmless because of its low potency, it may also be ineffective at treating a disorder. This is why it is important to work in conjunction with a trained homeopathic physician. It might be prudent to utilize a combination remedy that has been worked out for a specific diagnosis and proven over time to help.

Homeopathy and the Eyes

Good eyecare professionals realize that the eyes respond to nutritional influences and environmental factors, as all integral parts of the body do. There are many possible remedies for each eye condition. There are not, however, very many homeopathic remedies specifically for the numerous and varied eye disorders that can afflict people. It must be noted that most of the recommendations here may be considered general—that is, prescribed for a general underlying condition that results in eye symptoms. The remedy may not be directed at the specific eye disorder, or even at the chief complaint, but at the person as a whole. The correct remedy may act instantaneously, like an electric spark, upon the defense mechanism or vital force, and the effects of one dose may last as long as one month.

Homeopathic remedies may take the form of pellets, tablets, creams, oral liquids, or topical eye drops. The oral liquid type is an alcohol-based extract of a specific remedy, and therefore should not be used directly on the eye. The liquid is generally placed under the tongue with an eyedropper, which usually comes with the bottle. The liquid can also be used to make a cream, ointment, or salve, which is done by mixing with a cream or gel base. Creams, ointments, and salves are almost never used on eye tissue itself. Tablets and pellets are made with a base of lactose (sweet milk sugar) and dissolved in the mouth, usually under the tongue, without chewing. They are excellent for use with children. They should not, however, be touched, as doing so may decrease effectiveness. For infants, dissolve a pellet or tablet in water and administer it to the child using an eyedropper. Since oral liquid remedies contain alcohol, they should be given to children only in small doses.

The best time to take a homeopathic treatment is a few minutes before or thirty minutes after eating. Homeopathy requires personal observation to determine length of treatment. If no change occurs in a chronic ailment after a week, switch to another remedy. If improvement is noted, continue with the remedy until all symptoms disappear. It is very important to be aware of symptoms because the remedy should change as symptoms change. For example, a sore throat may turn into a headache, which may turn into sneezing or coughing, which may lead to a runny nose. Each of these symptoms has a separate remedy that is specific for that symptom. Review the previous table for specific eye-related remedies.

As mentioned, homeopathic treatment is unique and differs from traditional Western medicine. Homeopathic remedies treat a series of symptoms as unique, without necessarily assigning them a syndrome name. You may be tempted to treat your symptoms based on the conditions listed in this book and the remedies given for each. A homeopathic practitioner, however, may see a whole other set of symptoms based on further questioning, which may indicate the need for a different remedy. A homeopath will take a patient's physical characteristics and emotional state into consideration. It is best to consult a trained homeopathic practitioner before attempting any treatment.

DRUG-NUTRIENT INTERACTION

When filling out case history forms, many patients seem to forget about their vitamin or mineral supplements. Most people do not think to mention a vitamin or mineral supplement when asked about any medications they might be taking. They may consider this information inconsequential, or they may actively hide it from their doctors. It seems contradictory, but most people do not factor nutritional supplements into health status.

Treating nutritional supplements casually or keeping them a secret from a physician could be a big mistake. Some medications are known to interact with minerals or vitamins in a negative way. The popularity of vitamin and mineral supplements has increased dramatically over the past decade, as baby boomers look to remain healthy. With over half the

American population taking vitamins, the potential for problematic interactions with popular drugs is considerable.

Unfortunately, researchers have not devoted enormous amounts of time and energy to the study of how nutrients interact with drugs, partly because practical benefits of doing so would not be immediately apparent. The FDA has not required drug companies to spend the time or resources required to uncover negative interactions. The following chart summarizes information on how drugs affect nutritional status, and how nutritional supplements may interfere with drug benefits. This field is still evolving, and you should expect more information to become available over the next several years. Please remember to tell your practitioner about your supplement intake.

DRUG-NUTRIENT INTERACTION GUIDE		
Drug	**Nutrient**	**Interaction**
Accutane	Vitamin A	Because Accutane is related to vitamin A, taking these two compounds together could increase toxicity.
Antacids	Calcium phosphate Vitamin B_1 (thiamine)	The aluminum and magnesium in antacids can form a complex with phosphate and deplete the body of calcium. Aluminum-based antacids may inactivate thiamine. Do not take at mealtime.
Arthritis medicine (analgesics)	Iron Vitamin B_9 (folic acid) Vitamin C	Aspirin may block vitamin C absorption. Folic acid levels are lower in people who rely on large doses of aspirin. Small amounts of blood are regularly lost from the stomach when aspirin is taken. This can deplete the body of iron over time.
Birth control pills	Vitamin B_6 Vitamin B_9 (folic acid) Vitamin C Vitamin E	Women using combination oral contraceptives may need more of these B vitamins and vitamin E. Vitamin C, however, may increase blood levels of estrogen.
Blood pressure medicine	Potassium	Popular blood pressure medications tend to maximize potassium levels. This is fine unless the person is getting extra potassium through a potassium supplement or a potassium-based salt substitute.

Drug	Nutrient	Interaction
Blood thinners	Fish oil Vitamin C Vitamin E Vitamin K	Fish oil has blood-thinning effects, but research has shown that moderate amounts can be safely used with blood thinners. Very large amounts of vitamin C (5 g or more) could interfere with the effectiveness of blood thinners. The combination of Vitamin E and blood thinners thins the blood too much, leading to bruising or excessive bleeding. Vitamin K makes blood thinners less effective.
Broad-spectrum antibiotics	Vitamin K	Broad-spectrum antibiotics can destroy the intestinal bacteria that make vitamin K, which may lead to unusual bleeding.
Cholesterol medicine (statins)	Vitamin A Vitamin B_9 (folic acid) Vitamin B_{12} Vitamin D Vitamin E Vitamin K	This medication can interfere with absorption of fat and fat-soluble vitamins. Some studies suggest that vitamin D and even iron absorption may also be adversely affected. Because of their impact on vitamin K, these drugs could cause complications in combination with blood thinners. Blood tests are advised. All vitamins should be taken at a different time than the medication.
Corticosteroids	Calcium Potassium Vitamin D_3 Vitamin B_6 Vitamin B_9 (folic acid) Vitamin B_{12}	Cortisone-like drugs can deplete the body of vitamin D_3, vitamin B_6, vitamin B_{12}, folic acid, and potassium. They may also interfere with calcium absorption and metabolism. Long-term use may result in bone loss.
Diuretics	Calcium Magnesium Potassium	Diuretics may cause the loss of important minerals from the body. Periodic blood tests are essential to see whether supplements are needed.
Epilepsy drugs	Calcium Vitamin B_6 Vitamin B_9 (folic acid) Vitamin D	Folic acid and vitamin B_6 supplements can reduce blood levels of this anticonvulsant, potentially leading to seizures. If supplementation is needed, it should be carefully monitored. Barbiturates such as phenobarbital interfere with metabolism of vitamin D, leading to calcium loss.
Fluoro-quinolone	Calcium Iron Zinc	This type of antibiotic may not work as well as expected if taken at the same time as these minerals.

Drug	Nutrient	Interaction
Hormone replacement therapy	Vitamin B$_6$ Vitamin B$_9$ (folic acid) Vitamin E	Women using estrogen replacement therapy may need more of these vitamins. Too little vitamin B$_6$ could result in depression.
Indomethacin	Iron	Indomethacin irritates the stomach lining, even more so than aspirin. The continued low-level blood loss could lead to iron deficiency.
Laxatives	Vitamin A Vitamin D Vitamin E Vitamin K	Regular use of a mineral oil laxative interferes with proper absorption of the fat soluble vitamins. Lack of vitamin D can affect calcium and phosphate balance, and bone loss can occur.
Levodopa	Vitamin B$_6$	Vitamin B6 can reduce the effectiveness of this anti-Parkinson's disease drug. Supplementation should be avoided.
Methotrexate	Beta-carotene Vitamin B$_9$ (folic acid) Vitamin B$_{12}$	Methotrexate affects the intestinal wall, decreasing absorption of these nutrients.
Penicillin	Iron Copper Magnesium Vitamin B$_6$ Zinc	Penicillin may not be well absorbed if taken at the same time as iron or magnesium. It may also deplete the body of copper or zinc, causing a loss of the sense of taste.
Tagamet Zantac	Vitamin C Vitamin E	One theory suggests that reducing stomach acid could allow carcinogenic bacteria to survive in the stomach, increasing the risk of stomach cancer. These nutrients may protect the stomach.
Tetracycline	Calcium Iron Magnesium Vitamin B$_2$ (riboflavin) Vitamin C Zinc	These substances can combine with tetracycline so that the antibiotic is not absorbed properly. Avoid both antacids and supplements within two hours of a tetracycline pill. Long-term use of tetracycline may deplete these nutrients.
Thyroid hormone	Calcium Iron	Iron supplements taken at the same time as thyroid replacement hormone can reduce thyroid hormone effectiveness. Calcium may also interfere with levothyroxine absorption. Take these pills at least four hours apart.

Drug	Nutrient	Interaction
Tranquilizers	Vitamin B_2 (riboflavin) Vitamin B_{12} Vitamin C	Tranquilizers may deplete the body of riboflavin and vitamin B_{12}. A high dose of vitamin C may reduce the serum level of this type of drug.
Ulcer medication	Vitamin B_{12}	These acid-suppressing drugs can reduce absorption of vitamin B_{12} and chemically bind to protein. These effects may depend upon dose, and seem to disappear upon discontinuation of use.
Urinary anti-infectives	Vitamin B_9 (folic acid)	Medication for urinary tract infection interferes with folic acid metabolism. Folic acid deficiencies are unusual, however, as these drugs are usually prescribed for less than two weeks. If used for a longer period of time, supplementation may be warranted.

Before starting a pharmaceutical drug regimen to treat a health problem, always tell your healthcare practitioner about any supplements you are taking.

NUTRIENT-NUTRIENT INTERACTION

When people think of pharmaceuticals, they are generally confident that each drug is meant to target a specific site of action. There may be interaction between drugs, but each drug is given for a specific purpose, and many other drugs are often prescribed to counteract side effects. When considering a nutritional supplement or a particular food, there are numerous vitamins and minerals involved, and these nutrients usually interact with each other. Typically, a food isn't eaten because of only one nutrient it contains. All types of food have a varied complex of vitamins, minerals, and other substances that make them effective as fuel for the body.

The following section is designed as a guide to some of the interactions between nutrients, letting you know which nutrients affect others. Some interactions are positive and some are negative, so be sure to read each one carefully.

NUTRIENT-NUTRIENT INTERACTION GUIDE		
Nutrient	**Nutrient**	**Interaction**
Vitamin A	Vitamin C	Protect vitamin A from oxidation.
	Vitamin E	

Nutrient	Nutrient	Interaction
	Zinc	Required for metabolism of vitamin A and its transformation into active form.
	Calcium	Excessive vitamin A might affect calcium absorption.
Vitamin B$_3$ (niacin)	Choline	May reduce choline levels.
Vitamin B$_9$ (folic acid)	Zinc	Inhibits absorption of vitamin B$_9$.
	Vitamin C	Promotes conservation of vitamin B$_9$ in tissue.
	Vitamin B$_{12}$	Excess folic acid can mask a B$_{12}$ deficiency.
Vitamin C	Selenium	Selenium makes vitamin C more bioavailable.
Vitamin E	Vitamin C	Restores oxidized vitamin E.
	Selenium	Strengthens antioxidant properties.
Calcium	Vitamin D	Increases bioavailability of calcium.
	Magnesium	Converts vitamin D into its active form, supporting calcium absorption.
	Zinc	Excess reduces absorption of calcium.
Chromium	Iron	Reduces absorption of chromium.
Copper	Zinc	Excess reduces absorption of copper.
Iron	Calcium Zinc	Reduce absorption of iron.
	Vitamin A	Increases absorption of iron.
	Vitamin C	Increases absorption of iron.
Magnesium	Vitamin B$_6$	Promotes absorption and retention of magnesium.
	Calcium	Enhances absorption of magnesium.
	Vitamin D	Magnesium converts vitamin D into its active form, supporting calcium absorption.
Manganese	Calcium Iron	Impair absorption of manganese.
Molybdenum	Copper	Excess reduces absorption of molybdenum.

Nutrient	Nutrient	Interaction
Zinc	Vitamin B$_9$ (folic acid)	Inhibits absorption of zinc.
	Calcium Copper Iron	Reduce absorption of zinc in the intestine.
	Vitamin B$_2$ (riboflavin)	Increases bioavailability of zinc.

Considering the interactions that nutrients have with each other, a full-spectrum multivitamin formula from a reputable source may offer the best option for people looking to supplement their diets in a straightforward, easy-to-manage way.

NUTRIENT DEPLETION

Healthcare practitioners always have to be concerned with drug combinations due to the possible interaction of one drug with another. Considering that the average American over sixty years old takes at least eight or more medications, this is a very real issue. What some doctors fail to consider, however, is the way in which pharmaceutical drugs can affect nutrient levels in the body. Certain medications can inhibit absorption of vitamins, minerals, or other important substances. When specific nutrients remain depleted over time, various states of illness may result. As nutrients play a significant role in ocular health, these developments are worth noting. The following is a list of various drugs and the nutrients that are depleted through their usage, as well as the possible consequences of these combinations.

NUTRIENT DEPLETION GUIDE		
Medication	Nutrient Depleted	Possible Result
ACE inhibitors	Zinc	Loss of sex drive, infection, prostate problems, loss of sense of smell or taste, hair loss, slow wound healing, frequent infections, increased risk of cancer.

Medication	Nutrient Depleted	Possible Result
Acid Blockers	Almost all nutrients	Heart disease, high homocysteine, fatigue, Candida, cancer, irritable bowel, poor vision, high blood pressure.
Albuterol	Potassium	Irregular or rapid heartbeat, bone loss, confusion, muscle weakness, thirst, leg cramps.
Antibiotics	B vitamins	Heart disease, high homocysteine, fatigue, Candida, irritable bowel, increased risk of cancer.
Antipsychotics Major sedatives	CoQ_{10} Vitamin B_2 (riboflavin) vitamin B_{12}	Heart disease, high homocysteine, fatigue, headaches, insomnia, nerve pain, muscle ache, numbness, confusion, memory loss, Candida.
Aspirin	Vitamin B_5 Vitamin B_9 (folic acid) Vitamin C Calcium Iron	Fatigue, depression, osteoporosis, brittle nails, hair loss, edema, high cholesterol, homocysteine, heart disease, high blood pressure.
Beta blockers	CoQ_{10}	Heart disease, irregular heartbeat, memory loss, muscle cramps, insomnia, disrupted sleep, increased risk of cancer.
Blood pressure medication	CoQ_{10}	Fatigue, weakness, muscle and leg cramps, memory loss, increased risk of cancer, increased risk of infection, liver damage, increased risk of heart attack.
Calcium-channel blockers	CoQ_{10} Potassium	Irregular or rapid heartbeat, bone loss, confusion, muscle weakness, thirst, leg cramps.
Digoxin	Calcium Magnesium Phosphorus Vitamin B_1	Memory loss, muscle weakness, ankle swelling, depression, irritability, asthma, tooth decay, arrhythmias.
Dulcolax	Potassium	Irregular or rapid heartbeat, bone loss, confusion, muscle weakness, thirst, leg cramps.
Fibrates	Vitamin B_{12} Zinc	Heart disease, high homocysteine, fatigue, Candida, increased risk of cancer, irritable bowel, infection, hair loss, muscle pain, weakness, cramps, insomnia, vision problems.

Medication	Nutrient Depleted	Possible Result
Glyburide	CoQ_{10}	Fatigue, weakness, muscle cramps, memory loss, increased risk of cancer, infection, liver damage, heart disease.
HIV drugs	Copper Iron Zinc	Fatigue, anemia, liver problems, heart disease, blood sugar problems, loss of smell or taste.
Indomethacin	Iron Vitamin B_9 (folic acid)	Heart disease, high homocysteine, anemia, dermatitis, weakness, cervical dysplasia, depression, fatigue.
MAO inhibitors	Vitamin B_6	Heart disease, nerve pain, depression, mouth sores, fatigue, PMS, insomnia, dermatitis, fatigue.
Metformin	CoQ_{10} Vitamin B_9 (folic acid) Vitamin B_{12}	Heart disease, high homocysteine, infection, fatigue, anemia, irregular heartbeat, memory loss, increased risk of cancer, muscle cramps.
Methotrexate	Vitamin B_9 (folic acid)	Cervical dysplasia, increased risk of cancer, fatigue, depression, heart disease, nerve pain.
Mineral oil	Beta-carotene Calcium Magnesium Vitamin A Vitamin D Vitamin E Vitamin K	Heart disease, high homocysteine, fatigue, Candida, cancer, irritable bowel, increased risk of cancer, poor vision, high blood pressure.
NSAIDs	Vitamin B_9 (folic acid)	Heart disease, high homocysteine, cervical dysplasia, increased risk of cancer, risk of birth defects, depression.
Oral contraceptives	B vitamins Magnesium Selenium Zinc	Heart disease, fatigue, Candida, increased risk of stroke and cancer, irritable bowel, depression, insomnia, weakened immunity, memory loss, irritability, nerve pain, fatigue, low thyroid, inability to cope.
Phenytoin	B vitamins (especially vitamin B_9) Calcium Vitamin D Vitamin K	Anemia, fatigue, memory loss, depression, high homocysteine, heart problems, cervical dysplasia, increased risk of cancer.

Medication	Nutrient Depleted	Possible Result
Primidone	Vitamin B_9 (folic acid)	Anemia, high homocysteine, heart disease, hair loss, brittle nails, depression, skin problems, dermatitis.
Statins	CoQ_{10}	Fatigue, weakness, muscle cramps, memory loss, shortness of breath, increased risk of cancer, increased risk of infection, liver damage, heart disease.
Steroids (prednisone)	Calcium Potassium, most minerals Vitamin B_9 (folic acid) Vitamin C Vitamin D	Infection, osteoporosis, hearing loss, heart disease, fatigue, diabetes, slow wound healing, depression, irritability, weakness, birth defects, anemia, loss of sex drive, irritability.
Thyroid medication	Iron	Anemia, weakness, brittle nails, irritability, fatigue.

Always be sure to talk to your doctor about the ways in which nutrients or any other crucial compounds may be depleted from your body as a result of prescribed medication.

THE NEED FOR SUPPLEMENTS

In your quest to achieve not only eye health but also general health, do you need nutritional supplements or just a new diet? While most people like to think they can get their proper nutrition from food, doing so isn't easy in today's hectic, fast-paced world. The general supermarket has artificial and nutrient-poor food that lacks the basic nutrients needed on a daily basis. And then there is the junk food, which contains artificial ingredients that the human body may not even recognize. So, yes, you likely do need to supplement. Even the American Medical Association now recommends a full-spectrum multivitamin supplement for most individuals, especially if you are over the age of fifty.

Taking a full-spectrum supplement, eating real food (meaning almost no packaged food), and getting exercise are the best investments you can make in both short-term and long-term health. Farming food from overworked soil, processing it, storing it, and overcooking it are just a few of the ways food loses a large amount of its nutritional value. In reality, practical needs have outstripped the ability of even the very best diet to provide the nutrients required for great health. A high-quality multivitamin supplement should be the foundation of every nutrition program. Despite all the research proving the efficacy of supplements in preventing disease and promoting optimal health, too many physicians still don't take them seriously because they are too busy to read micronutrient studies published in nutrition and biochemistry journals. A large amount of published scientific evidence suggests a full-spectrum multivitamin supplement is good insurance, and could markedly improve health for those who consume inadequate diets, which is the majority of people in the United States. For example, the National Health and Nutrition Examination Survey (NHANES) assessed the health and nutritional status of adults and children in the United States, collecting detailed information about food, nutrient, and supplement intake, as well as other dietary behaviors. According to this survey, over 22 percent of respondents said they consumed fruit and vegetables more than five times a day, but a further review of the statistics showed that the percentage was actually closer to 10 percent.

RDA VS OPTIMAL HEALTH

The Food and Nutrition Board at the National Academy of Science sets the Recommended Daily Allowance or Daily Value at minimal levels needed to prevent diseases such as scurvy and rickets, not at levels that support optimal health. With the aging of the population, it has become popular to maintain a healthy lifestyle in an effort to slow the effects of age. Unfortunately, low-potency multivitamins and cheap formulations don't supply the right levels or proper balance of vitamins and minerals.

Every cell in the human body derives nutrients from food or supplements, which are carried to them via the bloodstream. The semipermeable membrane that surrounds each cell allows only a select number of micronutrients to cross its barrier. Minerals are also controlled by signaling factors in the membrane of the cell. Each nutrient must be transported to the site of its action by lipoproteins. Long-term consumption of excessively high amounts of any single nutrient may cause a deficiency of another nutrient in the body. If there is an excess of a water-soluble nutrient, the body will simply excrete it in the urine or sweat. Fat-soluble vitamins, however, are more difficult to excrete. Needless to say, the body's cells require sufficient amounts of nutrients, and in proper balance, to manage metabolism adequately.

HOW TO CHOOSE SUPPLEMENTS

When considering a supplement, it is important to know how well it is absorbed. Powdered supplements in vegetable capsule form are more easily broken down during digestion than pressed pills. In general, absorption rate is associated with both the quality and cost of the raw ingredient. Typically, inexpensive one-a-day products tend to have lower absorption rates than high-quality powdered formulations. Multivitamins should be taken at least twice a day with meals. Any one-a-day pill will not allow nutrients to be absorbed in proper balance. The human body uses water-soluble micronutrients as it needs them, and any extra is normally excreted within hours. Therefore, these essential micronutrients should be replenished at least twice a day. Conversely, fat-soluble vitamins are stored in the liver and slowly released as needed for proper metabolic function.

You should look for supplements that include balanced amounts of the full-spectrum of vitamins, including the vitally important B complex. Additionally, they should include the full spectrum of minerals, including trace minerals. Minerals are vital to the production of certain biochemicals that send messages to the nervous system, thyroid, and adrenal glands. These messages are involved in the production of hormones as well as in the efficient burning of calories.

Opt for supplements with plant-based antioxidants. Antioxidants help neutralize free radicals, which are associated with a number of chronic degenerative diseases, including diseases of the eye. It is important to note, however, that xanthophyll, an antioxidant related to macular health, is rarely included in supplement formulations, and when it is included, it is normally for marketing purposes only and in amounts far less than used in most micronutrient studies.

While supplements may promote growth and repair of the body, they cannot compete with double cheeseburgers and milkshakes. A good diet with an adequate amount of fruit and vegetables is the proper starting point for healthful living.

Conclusion

When discussing nutrition and supplements with your doctor, you should feel confident in your nutritional education. While you may consider yourself well educated in many areas of health, nutritional education is a specialized area in which most people lack proper knowledge. The real challenge is to find authentic nutritional information that is not either misleading or specifically sponsored by a commercial interest.

In learning about the science of nutrition, it is important to consider how nutritional research is conducted and how it differs from the randomized clinical trial (RCT) method, which is the gold standard for pharmaceutical research. All scientists recognize RCTs because they are such an important piece of the research puzzle in regard to drug testing, but you should not ignore other forms of research. Case-control and cohort studies, authentic meta-analyses, and other epidemiological data often indicate where further research should be focused, and they may prove or disprove hypotheses as well as develop them. In fact, RCTs are poorly suited to the evaluation of nutritional effects for several reasons. First, chronic diseases generally have long latencies and multifactorial causations, making it difficult to determine exactly how long a disease has been developing. Without knowing the starting point of an illness, it is difficult to know when certain treatments may be effective.

Unlike drugs, nutrients can have beneficial effects on multiple body tissues and interact in a dynamic fashion with other nutrients found in supplements and diet. Most RCTs, however, can test only one or two compounds, each at a single dose over a few years. This is too short a period to have significant impact on chronic degenerative disease, which can take decades to develop. All food contains a variety of nutritional ingredients designed to work synergistically. We don't eat spinach just because it contains lutein, for example. Nutrients act in helpful ways in virtually every body system; drugs act only on single targets potentially.

It is crucial to look at the full spectrum of micronutrient research and evidence available, including observational studies, because it can provide a clearer picture of the benefits of supplements. Observational studies can often better represent typical populations. These studies have a closer relationship to how foods and supplements are used in the real world. Additionally, observational studies are typically the only ethical approach in cases where eliminating essential nutrients as part of the study's design could be detrimental to the study's population. For an observational study there is the absence of a "no exposure" group. One cannot require subjects in a study not to take a specific nutritional product for an extended period of time. For example, you could not ask one group of participants to avoid vitamin C for several years simply to note the results of such a drastic lifestyle modification.

When it comes to vision health, you should review products by companies who specialize in supplements for eyecare needs. Products should have current valid scientific rationales available for anyone to review, as well as websites that puts science first before price and marketing. In addition, these companies should be third-party current Good Manufacturing Practices (cGMP) certified. Some authorities suggest that nutrients be purchased only from large manufacturers, but consider that these big companies are less likely to make an alteration in their formulations when updated science emerges. When a company has several thousands of dollars tied up in on-the-shelf product, it is extremely costly to remove that product for an updated version. Smaller companies have much more flexibility in this regard.

Be wary of store-brand nutritional supplements. Many times the store that purchases them has little or no say in their quality or ingredients. Also be cautious when shopping for supplements at large outlet warehouse stores that sell items in bulk. Sometimes these pills can sit in their bottles for several months, or even a year or more, if not purchased quickly enough. Many of the ingredients can become rancid long before those lengths of time.

The area of nutritional support for eye health is rapidly growing and emerging science is discovering more and more reasons for patients to take nutritional supplements. The information in this book combined with proper counseling from your primary eyecare practitioner can help you to see clearly well into your later years. Simply taking a few vitamins, however, will not overcome the detrimental effects of a poor diet. You need to alter your lifestyle overall to ensure not only healthy eyes but also a healthy life.

Index